T0234700

# Lecture Notes in Bioengineering

Lecture Notes in Bioengineering (LNBE) publishes the latest developments in bioengineering. It covers a wide range of topics, including (but not limited to):

- Bio-inspired Technology & Biomimetics
- Biosensors
- Bionanomaterials
- Biomedical Instrumentation
- Biological Signal Processing
- Medical Robotics and Assistive Technology
- Computational Medicine, Computational Pharmacology and Computational Biology
- Personalized Medicine
- Data Analysis in Bioengineering
- Neuroengineering
- Bioengineering Ethics

Original research reported in proceedings and edited books are at the core of LNBE. Monographs presenting cutting-edge findings, new perspectives on classical fields or reviewing the state-of-the art in a certain subfield of bioengineering may exceptionally be considered for publication. Alternatively, they may be redirected to more specific book series. The series' target audience includes advanced level students, researchers, and industry professionals working at the forefront of their fields.

Indexed by SCOPUS, EI Compendex, INSPEC, zbMATH, SCImago.

More information about this series at http://www.springer.com/series/11564

Mowafa Househ · Elizabeth Borycki ·
Andre Kushniruk
Editors

# Multiple Perspectives on Artificial Intelligence in Healthcare

Opportunities and Challenges

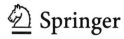 Springer

*Editors*
Mowafa Househ
College of Science and Engineering
Division of Information and Computing
Technology
Hamad Bin Khalifa University
Doha, Qatar

Elizabeth Borycki
Health Information Science
University of Victoria
Victoria, BC, Canada

Andre Kushniruk
Health Information Science
University of Victoria
Victoria, BC, Canada

ISSN 2195-271X          ISSN 2195-2728   (electronic)
Lecture Notes in Bioengineering
ISBN 978-3-030-67305-5       ISBN 978-3-030-67303-1   (eBook)
https://doi.org/10.1007/978-3-030-67303-1

This Springer imprint is published by the registered company Springer Nature Switzerland AG
The registered company address is: Gewerbestrasse 11, 6330 Cham, Switzerland

# Preface

Artificial intelligence (AI) in health care has garnered considerable interest in recent years. AI refers to a wide range of computer systems and applications that can be said to exhibit intelligence through use of a variety of technological innovations. Reports of use of AI to aid in the diagnosis, treatment and management of a wide number of healthcare conditions and diseases are being reported at an increasing rate in both the scientific literature and the media. In addition, AI applications are making their way to the general public, with new applications designed to aid with health promotion with the objective of making citizens healthier through use of advanced technology. AI is also being used to improve the effectiveness and efficiency of healthcare delivery (e.g. to address emergency room wait times). Application areas now range from use in dermatology to identify malignant skin cancers to use in robotic surgery and internal medicine, as well as cancer treatment and healthcare delivery management. Many of these advances in healthcare AI applications have been impressive, such as the increased use and reliance in practice on machine learning for processing radiological images.

Although the recent strong and renewed attention on AI in health care has led to considerable interest by both the public and the scientific communities, the application of AI to health care has had a long, extensive and at times tenuous history. This began with some of the earliest AI expert systems in the 1970s, through to application of neural nets in health care, to more recent advances in deep learning systems and biomedical data mining applications across a range of medical and health areas. In addition, AI is beginning to become more closely integrated into virtual and remote healthcare services. Along the way, there have been many reported successes. However, going back to the earliest applications through to today, the widespread dissemination of these technologies has met with a number of roadblocks, barriers and challenges. Indeed, many of these applications did not move past the stage of prototype or demonstration system. It is interesting to note that a number of recurring issues persist that were encountered during earlier iterations of AI research and application in health care. For example, challenges around testing and ensuring the validity of clinical decisions made by AI, determining the most effective ways of integrating such systems into healthcare workflow, as well as a range of logistical, safety, regulatory, ethical and policy issues, have accompanied many of the technical advances that have been achieved. An underlying motivation of this book is to consider both the successes of AI in health care, but also to address some previous as well as new and emerging challenges to bringing the full potential of this technology to bear on improving human health and well-being.

What makes this book unique is that it examines both the opportunities and challenges in applying AI methods, tools and technologies within health care from a number of different perspectives. The book covers several areas including: (1) human, management and policy perspectives and challenges for AI in health care, (2) AI challenges from the health professional perspective and (3) both advances and challenges from technological perspectives related to topics ranging from machine learning to text mining. Several of the papers focus on topics related to the human factors of AI in health care from a broad perspective. This includes considering issues around how to integrate AI into healthcare practices as well as ensuring both the effectiveness and safety of these new technologies. Other important aspects covered include privacy, trust and policy issues and challenges, which have become critical areas for understanding if AI is to become accepted and integrated into mainstream healthcare practice and education. Another group of papers in this book focuses on AI from the perspective of the health professional, including the increasing impact of AI on pharmacy and other professional areas such as use of natural language for chat bots in mental health. A further focus is on the advances in the area of machine learning and data mining in health care. This section of the book includes reviews and critiques of deep learning in health care, reinforcement learning applications and deep learning in biomedical text mining.

The book is designed to provide health scientists, data scientists, computer scientists, healthcare professionals, healthcare managers and policy-makers with insight into some of the key challenges and opportunities of AI in health care. The book is designed to challenge some of the preconceptions around AI in health care and to stimulate a pragmatic and balanced discussion about both some of the success of AI in health care and some challenges and issues that will need to be addressed before AI can achieve its full potential in streamlining, modernizing and improving healthcare processes and outcomes. It is hoped some of the challenges posed in the book will challenge preconceptions, provide insight into what is possible and potentially derive new solutions and ideas to the challenges posed in the book.

Doha, Qatar                                                                                          Mowafa Househ
Victoria, Canada                                                                              Elizabeth Borycki
Victoria, Canada                                                                                  Andre Kushniruk

# Acknowledgements

We thank the efforts of Dr. Alaa A. Abd-Alrazaq, Raghad M. Muhiyaddin and Asma Hassan from Hamad Bin Khalifa University, College of Science and Engineering, for their help and support in communicating with the authors, reviewers and the publisher leading to the publication of this important work. We also would like to thank Professor Mounir Hamdi, Founding Dean, Hamad Bin Khalifa University, College of Science and Engineering, for providing Dr. Mowafa Househ with the time and support needed to complete this work. Finally, we would like to thank the University of Victoria, School of Health Information Science, for their continuous support for making this work possible.

# Contents

# AI From Human, Management and Policy Perspectives

# The Human Factors of AI in Healthcare: Recurrent Issues, Future Challenges and Ways Forward

**Andre Kushniruk and Elizabeth Borycki**

**Abstract** There is considerable interest and excitement around the application of artificial intelligence (AI) in healthcare. Indeed, there have been a range of successful systems employing methods from AI such as artificial neural nets, machine learning, natural language processing and deep learning approaches to diagnosis and treatment. As the number of AI applications continues to grow, issues and challenges around how to integrate the technology into actual healthcare practice need to be considered. Many of these issues center around a range of human factors. There is the need to design more effective and reliable interactions between human and machine in the context of AI. In this chapter we identify and discuss a range of issues, many of which predate the current interest in AI in healthcare. Potential approaches to overcoming these challenges are also discussed in the context of designing more effective interactions with human end users.

**Keywords** Human factors · Artificial intelligence · Healthcare · Usability · Health information systems

## 1 Introduction

Artificial Intelligence (AI) in healthcare has become an area of widespread interest. AI promises to improve and modernize the ways in which healthcare services are provided. Indeed, AI techniques and methods are already revolutionizing some specific areas of healthcare, for example automated radiographic image pre-processing and image interpretation. However, there are a number of areas in which the application of AI in healthcare, although of considerable interest and promise, has encountered barriers to adoption. It is becoming clear that certain barriers will need

---

A. Kushniruk (✉) · E. Borycki
School of Health Information Science, University of Victoria, Victoria, BC, Canada
e-mail: andrek@uvic.ca

E. Borycki
e-mail: emb@uvic.ca

© Springer Nature Switzerland AG 2021
M. Househ et al. (eds.), *Multiple Perspectives on Artificial Intelligence in Healthcare*,
Lecture Notes in Bioengineering, https://doi.org/10.1007/978-3-030-67303-1_1

to be overcome in order for AI approaches to become mainstream across healthcare systems.

In this chapter it will be argued that many of the issues encountered today are related to human factors aspects of automating healthcare processes currently carried out by humans. Indeed, considerations from the field of human computer interaction (HCI) continue to have considerable implications for success or failure of adoption of AI in healthcare. Furthermore, it will be argued that many of the issues are similar to those that were encountered historically in previous waves of AI research, enthusiasm and investment. Even though some of the underlying technologies have greatly advanced, many HCI issues persist today that date back several decades.

A closer consideration of these human factors related issues, in light of the more recent advances of AI in healthcare, could be important for ensuring that advances in AI are able to fully meet their potential to modernize healthcare processes and positively transform healthcare. It will be argued that although the technical approaches and methods of AI in healthcare have advanced rapidly, understanding how to integrate AI technology with human processes has lagged behind the technological advances and innovation.

## 2   A Brief History of Human Factors Issues in Healthcare AI

AI in healthcare has a long history and can be characterized as having gone through a number of cycles or phases. Early work on expert systems in medicine dates back to the 1970s (Shortliffe et al. 1975). This work led to a boom in research in advancing AI systems in areas including diagnostic decision-making, natural language processing, and knowledge representation (Nilsson 2014). Further advances in neural networks and approaches to symbolic processing also prospered in the 1980s and 1990s and have continued to today with major advances in areas such as machine learning, computer imaging and robotics (Russell and Norvig 2016). However, the road to advancement of AI in healthcare has not been a smooth one and has had many failed initiatives, with many reported issues having arisen in relation to end user acceptance. Furthermore, a number of barriers to integration of AI technology into mainstream healthcare practice have been encountered. Many of these human factors related issues have lingered over the years, despite the continual advancement of the technical methods used in AI applications themselves.

In a review of the fields of AI and HCI, the term "AI winter" has appeared to describe periods of downturn in funding and interest in AI, in contrast to other periods that have shown strong optimism (and funding) for AI—one such cycle, it could be argued, we are currently in. Interestingly, Grudin has argued that major advances and funding in HCI appear to have corresponded to periods that could be described as AI winters. This has led to some interesting speculations as to why this may have occurred, and why interests (and research funding) might shift between AI and human factors in what appears to be a cyclic pattern (Grudin 2009). In the history of AI in medicine, the period in the 1970s and 1980s led to considerable research in areas such as expert systems, natural language processing and the introduction of connectionist approaches such as neural networks (Buchanan 2005). Concomitant with this was the establishment of numerous research groups and centres focusing on AI in healthcare worldwide.

However, by 1990 it was acknowledged widely that much the promise of AI up to that point had not fully come to fruition (as evidenced by the large number of "prototype" systems developed with far fewer operational systems in practice), as the difficulty of implementing AI systems in healthcare was found to be greater than initially expected and considered. By 1990 Miller and Massarie (developers of the influential medical expert system known as Internist) reflected on this situation in a seminal paper entitled "The Demise of the "Greek Oracle" Model for Medical Diagnostic Systems" (Miller and Masarie 1990). Those authors argued that an initial focus on early medical AI (specifically expert systems) on replacing rather than supporting or facilitating medical decision making (essentially pointing to the need for improved user interaction) was one reason why such systems were not adopted widely in medical practice. They argued instead of replacing human decision making, that what healthcare professionals wanted were tools that supported and helped the health professional with their own natural decision making processes. Such tools would ideally act as decision making "catalysts" that could be better integrated into their actual work practices and decision making processes. Thus, one consequence of this argument was that greater emphasis is needed to be placed on improved human–computer interaction when it came to AI applications to provide decision support (Kushniruk 2001).

This work led some researchers to explore improved ways of integrating clinical decision support into healthcare work practices, an endeavor that has moved from a focus on AI in isolation to AI in the context of naturalistic decision making and workflow—i.e. into the world at the intersection of HCI and healthcare (Li et al. 2012). It has been argued that in order to successfully introduce AI into healthcare a better understanding of the natural processes of healthcare decision making would be needed. Further study of how natural and artificial processes could be better integrated would also be needed in order to lead to more successful and widespread implementation of many AI systems and applications. It is argued in this chapter that the challenge of integrating AI and HCI has remained to be more fully explored, particularly in healthcare. Further work along these lines is needed before AI will reach its potential for modernizing and improving healthcare.

## 3   Human Factors Issues and Challenges in Healthcare AI

From a historical perspective, a number of issues and challenges related to HCI have emerged and continue to appear in the literature on AI in medicine, and now healthcare more generally. These issues have become particularly apparent as AI applications in healthcare move from the clinical and hospital setting to the wider healthcare environment (including use by not only some healthcare professionals but also patients and lay people). Some of these issues could be summarized as the following:

- Issues and challenges in integrating AI applications with existing healthcare software, systems and human work practices

  - Integrating AI into human healthcare processes in an effective way has been a challenge for many types of AI applications. In particular, AI systems designed to serve as decision support for diagnosis and treatment must take into account health professional practices and human cognitive limitations (as well as how to integrate them into workflow processes). Issues around how to effectively integrate such systems into the daily work activities of busy health professionals arose early on with medical expert systems and has continued to be a challenge today. Even with more modern diagnostic systems such as IBM's Watson, the human factors of integrating this type of technology into organizations has been reported as being problematic and needing further exploration (Schmidt 2017).
  - Integration of AI systems into today's healthcare organization's complex digital ecosystem (that has grown in complexity over the past several decades) can also be a challenge. This includes integrating AI systems within large proprietary systems, such as hospital-wide electronic health record systems (Strickland 2019). The issues of interoperability and sharing of data across systems is one that can be problematic for all types of information technology in healthcare organizations. These issues have also been reported as being particularly problematic and barriers to bringing AI applications into routine healthcare practice.

- Issues around generalization of AI solutions and local context

  - One of the challenges of AI that arose early on was the issue of how generalizable AI solutions were when transported from the localities where they were developed and then moved to healthcare organizations in new regions. Historically, a number of AI systems that were found to work well within the environment(s) they were initially designed in were found to be far less effective (and in some cases less accurate) when used in new locations and regions (Musen et al. 2006). Here a range of human factors related to differences in practice patterns and cultural differences have been identified as potential underlying issues.

- Complexities involved in knowledge acquisition, validation and maintenance

  - An issue that has been problematic in early AI research was known as the "knowledge acquisition bottleneck", where the acquisition, maintenance and upkeep of knowledge and data used to drive AI systems was found to be more complex than anticipated (i.e. becoming labelled as being a "bottle-neck"). Early AI systems attempted to address this by development of knowledge acquisition subsystems. With the advent of neural networks and machine learning systems (which do not involve acquisition of knowledge in symbolic form), this issue still persists in new ways (Wagner 2006). Such AI systems may depend on the data they are trained on and some AI systems may be susceptible to biases in the input data and limitations in the training data sets. This has led to new types of issues limiting generalizability of some AI systems and the potential for bias. As a consequence, the maintenance, updating and verification of data, information and knowledge (e.g. knowledge embodied in clinical guidelines used to drive automated alerting and remaindering systems) persists as an issue in healthcare.

- Issues around need for common-sense reasoning and "world knowledge" to support reasoning at a deeper level when required

  - Historically, in the literature on AI there have been philosophical debates for decades about to what extent could AI systems embody and display "deep reasoning" capabilities (i.e. "strong AI"), which can include common sense reasoning using a broad base of knowledge of the world (Sharkey and Ziemke 2001). Indeed, many of the current successes of AI in healthcare are those that are in a very specific domain and where systems can be trained to perform on constrained inputs, with limited outputs (e.g. binary decisions regarding presence or absence of particular types of lesions). In other areas, the successful inclusion of natural language processors (such chat bots for supporting direct dialog with patients) will require systems that can function reliably outside of restricted domains of knowledge discourse and such advancements are yet to have been achieved.

- Issues around trust and potential liability

  - Perhaps one of the most critical issues today with regard to acceptance of AI technologies in healthcare practice is related to end users' trust of AI technology, along with concerns about liability and impact of potential error resulting from use of AI technologies. Indeed, issues around certification and regulatory approval of AI technologies, including FDA approval processes, have to come the fore as healthcare organizations grapple with deciding whether or not to include AI technologies into regular practice. Such concerns are due to issues related to system quality, organizational liability and current lack of clarity around need for regulatory approval for many AI applications in healthcare (He et al. 2019).

- Issues around human understanding, need for explanation capability and transparency about results and outcomes

  - This brings up HCI issues (that have existed since the early days of expert systems in healthcare) around how results from AI can be interpreted and validated at the human end. Specifically, understanding how human understandable explanations can be created will be important for engendering human trust in AI solutions. This will be a continuing issue with neural network applications (where data is represented by large numbers of interconnected nodes) and machine learning algorithms (applying advanced statistical analyses) as the issue of visualizing the results of AI computation in a human understandable and transparent way is itself a research area (Gunning and Aha 2019). Physicians will be reluctant to use AI if they do not understand it or it has not been tested and found to improve clinical outcomes.

- The need for effective HCI interaction modes and models

  - Issues exist around how embedded or ubiquitous an AI application should be in order to support healthcare work and practices. Possible modes of interaction range from consulting by humans, critiquing human decisions, automated alerting, augmenting human perception and extending physical access (e.g. robotic surgery). Some systems may run entirely in the background (i.e. ubiquitous), provide active alerting and reminding (direct extension of rule-based AI), and applying machine learning and knowledge discovery (Musen et al. 2006).

- Differences in errors and error mode type

  - Error is inevitable and both humans and AI systems will make errors. However, analysis and comparison of the differences between the type, severity, distribution and frequency of errors that humans make as compared to the errors AI systems make can be difficult. This can lead to problems in assessing system safety and asserting which type of system (human or AI) is more accurate or safe for carrying out a healthcare task, given these differences. Understanding the differences in error has significant importance for assessment of safety and trust in new systems (Price et al. 2019).

- Complexities in achieving the appropriate balance between human and machine interaction

  - The balance between human and machine performance in AI human interactions is a complex issue and remains to be further explored. Examples include complexities in designing user interactions for robotic surgery. Although this technology is revolutionizing surgery, system designers still have the issue of designing user interactions with the technology that have the "right" balance of control. This is the issue of deciding which tasks should be performed by humans, which tasks AI can be used to complement human performance, and which tasks can be completely replaced by AI (which is parallel to issues in aviation where there is a tight and critical balance between automation and manual human control in design of aircraft). Further work in understanding human-AI interaction and human–robot interaction (which is itself becoming an active area of research) will be needed (Goodrich and Schultz 2008).

## 4 Characteristics of Successful AI Applications in Healthcare

Despite the many challenges to successfully implementing AI into healthcare described in the previous sections of this chapter, there are a number of areas where AI in healthcare has advanced rapidly and appears to be already transforming healthcare. In order to understand adoption patterns of AI, it is of value to consider the characteristics and nature of those application areas where AI has been more readily adopted in practice. This can be useful in order to understand the essential aspects of AI systems that facilitate adoption from a human factors perspective.

In working towards classifying AI applications we may ask, in the context of human factors, what are the areas where AI seems to work best and end up getting adopted by healthcare organizations? Along these lines, we are currently working on developing a framework for characterising successful AI applications in healthcare. The following are some of the contexts, based on our preliminary analysis of the literature, in which AI applications appear to have led to successful adoption:

- Providing healthcare workers with data that cannot otherwise be obtained
- Providing overview of data for rapid decision making that would otherwise lead to human cognitive overload, or take too long for human processing
- Providing support for tedious or time-consuming administrative functions, documentation, storage, or transportation of data
- Providing processing support for large data streams that would overwhelm humans—e.g. big data analytics and machine learning
- Providing automated safety alerts and reminders, when integrated appropriately into healthcare workflow.

More generally, from a human factors perspective it appears AI will be adopted if the AI solution:

- Is proven to work properly and is accurate—Food and Drug Administration (FDA) and other regulatory approval is important, but alone is not sufficient to ensure adoption
- Is needed in the first place—it solves a problem
- Is deemed useful e.g. saves time, money or increases efficiency
- Produces outputs that are accurate and trustable
- Can do useful tasks not otherwise possible due to size of data and processing constraints
- Allows for more timely access to healthcare
- Is financially and organizationally feasible and advantageous
- Is usable—i.e. fits into daily and complex healthcare activities and workflow as seamlessly as possible.

Perhaps the most effective application of AI in healthcare today is in the area of AI to support image pre-processing and interpretation of images, including analysis of chest radiographs and classification of suspicious skin lesions in dermatological applications. From such application, we can see that AI applications to date that have achieved such success in adoption tend to include applications that work on well-defined tasks, particularly those that can be trained to make decisions about binary (or limited option) choices (e.g. if a lesion is benign or malignant). Indeed, a number of such applications have rivalled or even outperformed human physicians when head to head comparisons were conducted in a number of now well cited studies in the areas of radiology, dermatology and pathology (Lakhani and Sundaram 2017).

In addition, AI applications designed to support services in under-resourced areas show particular early promise, particularly in areas where human expertise is in short supply. For example, there is limited access to radiological expertise in some countries where tuberculosis is prevalent. In some projects in such countries AI systems have allowed X-rays to uploaded, analyzed and interpreted by AI systems with a high degree of accuracy (Buch et al. 2018).

Finally, aspects of AI expert systems and research in knowledge representation has had an important impact in the area of developing automated alert and reminding systems, integrated into electronic health records and driven by evidence-based guidelines. This is an area of decision support that has routinely become incorporated into electronic health record systems in daily use and hence has tended by some to now be outside of the realm of AI (a fate which successful approaches emerging from the area of AI achieve once the technology has become more "mainstream").

## 5   Discussion—Future Directions for Work in the Human Factors of AI

Adoption of AI systems and applications by humans in healthcare can be considered in the context of innovation of new technology more generally (e.g. within the framework of Rogers' Innovation of Diffusion model). Roger's model posits that there are different types of users of new technology that adopt the technology over time, from early adopters (who are pioneers) through to majority users and finally laggards (those who are last to adopt). In future work it will be useful to examine the human factors that will need to be considered as different groups of users of technology move over time through all phases in the model, from early adopters to late majority users etc. This is where research on the information needs of the different types of adopters of AI in healthcare will be needed and could help in facilitating more rapid adoption of these new information technologies for a wider range of health professionals.

More generally, the role of usability engineering and advances in user experience (UX) design will become more critical as more AI applications are developed and efforts and attempts to deploy them in healthcare organizations increase. For example, the authors have been involved in the development of a user-centered methodological approach to designing, testing and deploying AI applications (Li et al. 2012). This approach involves a multi-layered and sequenced approach to evaluating AI and decision support applications. In one study we applied three different methods in refining and integrating alerts, intelligent risk calculators and intelligent presentation of order set information, all embedded within an electronic record system. This involved an initial phase of laboratory-based usability testing, where clinicians were video recorded as they interacted with mock ups of prototypes for the integration of evidence-based guidelines for driving alerts (using usability testing methods adapted to low-cost rapid analyses conducted within an actual hospital setting). Based on this initial phase of testing, refinements were made and a second simulation phase involving observing clinicians' interactions with a virtual "digital" patient was undertaken in order to assess how the new guidelines and decision support tools affected actual clinical workflow. Based on this second phase, the integration of the new technology was optimized to take into account when and how often clinicians preferred the "triggering" of the automated decision support tools. Finally, a third phase was conducted of "near-live" system testing (under real and actual conditions and context of use) prior to widespread release of the system (Li et al. 2012). This methodical and staged approach to design, testing and implementation ended up resulting in a high level of adoption of the new technology by clinicians. It is argued that such an approach, linking laboratory testing and feedback with naturalistic analysis of AI applications, will be essential to move adoption of AI forward in healthcare (Kushniruk et al. 2013). Further work in applying a range of methods from human factors research will be needed in order to better understand interaction between humans and AI and will be a needed direction for advancing AI technologies in healthcare.

An additional and rapidly emerging issue from a human factors perspective will be the challenge of understanding the information and cognitive processing needs of an increasingly wider range of users of AI systems and applications, including patients. As AI applications move from being targeted to supporting health professionals to use by the wider population (including patients and lay people—e.g. the Babylon system (Burgess 2017; Oliver 2019)) the need for better understanding human information needs and information processing capabilities and limitations, will only become more important and critical.

In conclusion, AI in healthcare promises to have a profound impact on improving healthcare and healthcare processes. In this chapter a number of challenges from a human factors perspective have been outlined, many of which had precursors from previous generation of AI research. It is argued that further consideration of AI applications from a human factors perspective will be critical in order to achieve the potential benefits of AI technology, given the complexity of human–computer interaction in healthcare.

# References

Buch VH, Ahmed I, Maruthappu M (2018) Artificial intelligence in medicine: current trends and future possibilities. Br J Gen Pract 68(668):143–144
Buchanan BG (2005) A (very) brief history of artificial intelligence. AI Mag 26(4):53–53

Burgess M (2017) The NHS is trialling an AI chatbot to answer your medical questions. Wired UK (2017, January 5). Retrieved from https://www.wired.co.uk/article/babylon-nhs-chatbot-app

Goodrich MA, Schultz AC (2008) Human–robot interaction: a survey. Found Trends® Hum–Comput Interact 1(3):203–275

Grudin J (2009) AI and HCI: two fields divided by a common focus. AI Mag 30(4):48–48

Gunning D, Aha DW (2019) DARPA's explainable artificial intelligence program. AI Magazine 44

He J, Baxter SL, Xu J, Xu J, Zhou X, Zhang K (2019) The practical implementation of artificial intelligence technologies in medicine. Nat Med 25(1):30–36

Kushniruk AW (2001) Analysis of complex decision-making processes in health care: cognitive approaches to health informatics. J Biomed Inform 34(5):365–376

Kushniruk A, Nohr C, Jensen S, Borycki EM (2013) From usability testing to clinical simulations: bringing context into the design and evaluation of usable and safe health information technologies. Yearb Med Inform 22(01):78–85

Lakhani P, Sundaram B (2017) Deep learning at chest radiography: automated classification of pulmonary tuberculosis by using convolutional neural networks. Radiology 284(2):574–582

Li AC, Kannry JL, Kushniruk A, Chrimes D, McGinn TG, Edonyabo D, Mann DM (2012) Integrating usability testing and think-aloud protocol analysis with "near-live" clinical simulations in evaluating clinical decision support. Int J Med Inform 81(11):761–772

Miller RA, Masarie FE Jr (1990) The demise of the "Greek Oracle" model for medical diagnostic systems. Methods Inf Med 29(01):1–2

Musen MA, Middleton B, Greenes RA (2006) Clinical decision-support systems. In: Shortliffe E, Cimino J (eds) Biomedical informatics in health care and biomedicine. Springer, Berlin

Nilsson NJ (2014) Principles of artificial intelligence. Morgan Kaufmann

Oliver D (2019) David Oliver: lessons from the Babylon Health saga. BMJ 365:l2387

Price WN, Gerke S, Cohen IG (2019) Potential liability for physicians using artificial intelligence. JAMA 322(18):1765–1766

Russell SJ, Norvig P (2016) Artificial intelligence: a modern approach. Pearson Education Limited, Malaysia

Schmidt C (2017) MD Anderson breaks with IBM Watson, raising questions about artificial intelligence in oncology. JNCI: J Nat Cancer Inst 109(5)

Sharkey NE, Ziemke T (2001) Mechanistic versus phenomenal embodiment: can robot embodiment lead to strong AI? Cogn Syst Res 2(4):251–262

Shortliffe EH, Davis R, Axline SG, Buchanan BG, Green CC, Cohen SN (1975) Computer-based consultations in clinical therapeutics: explanation and rule acquisition capabilities of the MYCIN system. Comput Biomed Res 8(4):303–320

Strickland E (2019) IBM Watson, heal thyself: how IBM overpromised and underdelivered on AI health care. IEEE Spectr 56(4):24–31

Wagner C (2006) Breaking the knowledge acquisition bottleneck through conversational knowledge management. Inform Resour Manage J (IRMJ) 19(1):70–83

# The Safety of AI in Healthcare: Emerging Issues and Considerations for Healthcare

**Elizabeth M. Borycki and Andre W. Kushniruk**

**Abstract**  In this book chapter we outline some of the emerging issues and considerations that will need to be considered by policy makers, clinicians, healthcare administrators, health technology developers, and implementers, when considering AI's use in the coming years. In addition to this, the authors propose a new framework for researching and evaluating the introduction of AI into clinical practice settings. We begin by discussing some of the challenges associated with implementing AI in healthcare. These challenges will need to be addressed in the near future as this technology moves towards being more widely used across varying healthcare contexts (e.g. physician office, community, hospital). Lastly, we propose a model for advancing future work in the area of AI in medicine and healthcare as a guide for addressing safety. We begin our chapter by defining AI and AI safety, followed by a review of some of the emerging issues and considerations for AI in healthcare.

## 1   Introduction

Artificial intelligence or AI has been touted as a potential solution for many healthcare problems from improving organizational efficiencies to enhancing human abilities to diagnose disease and identifying new treatments for chronic conditions such as cancers (Matheny et al. 2019; Price and Gerke 2019; Jiang et al. 2017; He et al. 2019). Even as AI is being considered as a potential radical advance to improving patient diagnosis and treatment, health professional performance and organizational work, there remain several issues associated with its safe use that need to be considered (Matheny et al. 2019; Price and Gerke 2019). A number of these issues are only beginning to be documented and discussed in the published literature as AI

E. M. Borycki · A. W. Kushniruk (✉)
School of Health Information Science, University of Victoria, Victoria, BC, Canada
e-mail: andrek@uvic.ca

E. M. Borycki
e-mail: emb@uvic.ca

© Springer Nature Switzerland AG 2021
M. Househ et al. (eds.), *Multiple Perspectives on Artificial Intelligence in Healthcare*,
Lecture Notes in Bioengineering, https://doi.org/10.1007/978-3-030-67303-1_2

technologies are tested and implemented in varying healthcare contexts (Matheny et al. 2019; Price and Gerke 2019; Jiang et al. 2017; He et al. 2019). In this book chapter we outline some of the emerging issues and considerations that will need to be considered by policy makers, clinicians, healthcare administrators, health technology developers, and implementers, when considering AI's use in the coming years. In addition to this, the authors propose a new framework for researching and evaluating the introduction of AI into clinical practice settings. We begin by discussing some of the challenges associated with implementing AI in healthcare. These challenges will need to be addressed in the near future as this technology moves towards being more widely used across varying healthcare contexts (e.g. physician office, community, hospital). Lastly, we propose a model for advancing future work in the area of AI in medicine and healthcare as a guide for addressing safety. We begin our chapter by defining AI and AI safety, followed by a review of some of the emerging issues and considerations for AI in healthcare.

## 2   What is AI?

AI in healthcare can be defined as the intersection between healthcare computing and health informatics. AI researchers and health informatics and health information technology professionals are designing, developing and implementing integrated computing and health informatics AI solutions designed to undertake tasks that are typically done by health professionals (e.g. diagnosing the presence of disease, recommending treatment approaches) and health administrators (e.g. managing wait times in an emergency department, effectively utilizing surgical resources in operating rooms) with greater speed, accuracy and efficiency (He et al. 2019). Several AI methods have been developed, tested and evaluated in healthcare over the past few decades. These methods include the application of neural networks and machine learning (e.g. reinforced learning, supervised learning and unsupervised learning) to health care problems and processes (Jiang et al. 2017; He et al. 2019; Brownlee 2019). It is during the application of these methods that researchers, policy makers and clinicians have identified several emerging issues and challenges that need to be considered for AI to be safely implemented in healthcare, and for administrators, clinicians and patients to trust the technology, when used to solve real-world healthcare problems. Such research is necessary to understand the subsequent impacts of implementing AI in healthcare (Matheny et al. 2019; Price and Gerke 2019; Jiang et al. 2017; He et al. 2019; Brownlee 2019). In the next section of the book chapter, the authors will outline the key emerging issues and challenges that have been identified by researchers, clinicians and administrators when implementing AI systems in medicine and healthcare.

# 3 Technology-Induced Errors in Healthcare and AI Safety

In 2005 several researchers found that there was a relationship between health technology features and functions and patient safety. These researchers found that in the programming, design, development, implementation and maintenance of health technologies, medical errors could inadvertently: (a) arise from the technology or (b) contribute to medical error thereby leading to a patient safety event. Researchers found a definitive relationship between medical errors and health technology features and functions (Kushniruk et al. 2005; Koppel et al. 2005). Health informatics researchers referred to this type of error as a technology-induced error (Kushniruk et al. 2005). Technology-induced errors can be "defined as those sources of error that arise from: (a) the design and development of technology, (b) the implementation and customization of a technology, and (c) the interactions between the operation of a technology and the new work processes that arise from a technology's use"(Borycki et al. 2012) as well as errors that arise when two systems interface to transmit and exchange data (Kushniruk et al. 2012). Technology-induced errors when left uncorrected could lead to significant medical errors across a healthcare system as they propagate through the system of care (Borycki et al. 2009). In subsequent follow-up studies from around the world focusing on patient safety incident reporting systems, researchers were able to link health technology events to incidents of patient death and disability (Magrabi et al. 2012; Palojoki et al. 2017). These works led to the development of a new field of research in health informatics and health information technology safety (Borycki et al. 2016). With the emergence of this area of research in health information technology and health informatics, theories, frameworks and methods were constructed, developed and tested to better understand how technology-induced errors emerge and how they can be prevented from occurring (Borycki et al. 2012; Borycki et al. 2016; Borycki and Keay 2010). AI, like other technologies, designed, developed and implemented for use in healthcare can introduce new types of errors (Matheny et al. 2019). These "new" or emerging technology-induced errors have their origins in aspects of the technology and the environments where the technology is deployed. In the next section of this book chapter, the authors will describe and outline these safety issues from a data safety, which may put the patients' private information in jeopardy, through to a patient safety, which may put the patient at harm or risk of death, perspective.

# 4 Data and Safety of AI Solutions

In order for robust AI solutions to be developed for clinical settings, large amounts of data are required to train AI systems, followed by access to an ongoing data supply to continue training, validating, and improving the AI system over time so that it is better able to detect potential disease, solve medical challenges and healthcare system problems (Matheny et al. 2019; Jiang et al. 2017; He et al. 2019). Such access is important to improve the quality and safety of the AI system (i.e. the ability of the AI solution to detect what it was designed to detect) (Matheny et al. 2019; Jiang et al. 2017; He et al. 2019; Kim et al. 2020). Training ensures that the technology can identify the presence and/or absence of disease (Kim et al. 2020). AI solutions may also be applied to healthcare processes such as improving healthcare staffing needs to meet the demand for services in areas such as the emergency room (Menke et al. 2014), and mining administrative data for insights that might help identify new methods of treating disease or suggesting a treatment for a disease (Bellini et al. 2019). Of note, in as much as there is an expectation that AI systems identify the presence or absence of disease or improve the efficiency of healthcare processes, there is also an expectation that the technology be effective in supporting relevant patient and/or healthcare processes to support decision making. Here, there is an expectation that systems do not miss important data that could lead to a medical error in decision-making (especially in the context of diagnosing disease) (Matheny et al. 2019; Price and Gerke 2019; He et al. 2019). For example, there have been documented health professional and consumer expectations that newly introduced algorithms consistently and accurately identify common through to rare health conditions to support the diagnosis of disease and to ensure that no errors are made by the technology. This is also important as there is a need to ensure that no undue negative impacts arise during physician decision making  (Matheny et al. 2019; Price and Gerke 2019; He et al. 2019).

## 5   Data, Safety and the Role of Large Datasets

To develop algorithms that can detect common and rare forms of disease consistently, large datasets are needed (Matheny et al. 2019; Kim et al. 2020). Large datasets can be difficult for a healthcare organization to collect, acquire and/or grow; for example, electronic health record data is among the most common types of data that are being considered by AI researchers for training and validating AI algorithms (He et al. 2019). Researchers have suggested access to such large repositories of data may be insufficient and due to their limited size, the data sets may be inadequate to fully train and validate an AI solution. Researchers have also indicated that in order to address the relative absence of large data sets, there may be a need to pool data across nations and healthcare organizations for adequate and effective algorithm testing and validation to take place (i.e. testing that ensures the quality and safety of algorithms) (He et al. 2019; Kim et al. 2020). To do this, large healthcare organizations and governments would need to develop technology products and infrastructures that are able to anonymize large patient data sets and to provide that data in a secure environment where the safety of that data is maintained and the privacy of individuals whose data is in the dataset is ensured (He et al. 2019; Kim et al. 2020).

# 6 Data, Safety, and Patient Privacy

Healthcare datasets with sensitive patient information provide researchers with opportunities to create AI solutions. Yet, healthcare organizations and governments need to ensure the safety and security of health data used for AI system development, testing and validation. There is a need for policy makers to modify legislative and regulatory requirements surrounding patient privacy and confidentiality to provide researchers and AI developers with access to that data in such a way as the safety and privacy of each person's data in that dataset is maintained. The safety of data is critical and needed to prevent security breaches and violations of patient confidentiality. Investment will need to be made by policy makers, governments and industry to ensure that data breaches and de-identification techniques are developed to protect the privacy of patients and to create legislation and develop regulatory requirements that protect the privacy and confidentiality of patients. Until such a time when large datasets become available, there is risk that AI systems using this data will not meet the quality and safety standards expected by administrators, clinicians and consumers of the technology to robustly detect the presence or absence of all forms of disease (Jiang et al. 2017; He et al. 2019).

# 7 Effects of Dataset Quality in Healthcare and Safety

Earlier in this chapter we identified the importance of robust data sets. Clinical relevancy of data is important and emerging issue in the development of AI. Here, it is necessary to identify the types of data that would be needed for training and validation to develop safe and effective AI. For example, Kim and colleagues (2020) conducted a retrospective multi-reader study with a focus on breast cancer detection. In their work they used data sets from institutions in three countries to obtain an ethically diverse data set. The mammography data were confirmed as: (1) cancer positive through biopsy, (2) benign by biopsy or follow-up imaging or (3) normal. The Kim study (2020) illustrates the importance of data sets that are robust in terms of the types of clinically relevant data that were selected to train the AI algorithm—mammography and biopsy data. The work draws attention to the use of relevant and high quality data in developing AI (Price and Gerke 2019; Jiang et al. 2017; He et al. 2019; Kim et al. 2020).

# 8 AI in Healthcare Contexts

AI, like other health technologies needs to be considered in the context of the technologies that are currently used in the healthcare system, such as electronic health records, diagnostic imaging systems, laboratory information systems and other digital solutions. There is a need to understand the ecosystem of technologies and how they "fit" together and where AI can be inserted, added or replaced to enhance clinician decision-making and improve workflow in healthcare organizations. When tied to these two areas of concern there is a need to assess the ability of AI to "fit" into work and to provide a benefit over and above existing technologies and systems of care. To illustrate, AI aimed at enhancing clinician decision making should be studied to determine, if it can improve a clinicians' diagnostic abilities in differing contexts and what supports will be needed (e.g. clinician, patient) to ensure the technology is used effectively and efficiently (Matheny et al. 2019; Price and Gerke 2019; He et al. 2019). Alternatively, from an organizational perspective, AI needs to be studied to determine if the technology can improve local processes such as helping to reduce emergency room wait times, AI systems to support patient monitoring and in other cases to enhance diagnosis of disease and treatment (due to the algorithms capacity to undertake activities previously done by clinicians) (Menke et al. 2014; Bellini et al. 2019). Key to this is the need to determine if the technology works and where it works best in the context of clinician and organizational workflows before the technology is implemented so that patient safety and quality of care are maintained (He et al. 2019; Menke et al. 2014; Bellini et al. 2019).

## 9    Research Evidence: How Do We Evaluate the Safety and Quality of AI?

There exists considerable debate in the computer science, health informatics, health services administration and the medical literature about the types of research evidence that will be needed to ensure that AI delivers on its promised expectations. There has recently emerged research in the health informatics, data science and computer science communities identifying that AI solutions' reproducibility is a focus of concern (Barber 2019). AI systems developed on one dataset do not necessarily have the same results when applied to other data sets. This has led to calls by researchers in the health informatics, data science and computer science communities for increased transparency, a research focus on AI reproducibility and AI testing on local datasets before the technology is fully implemented (He et al. 2019; Barber 2019). Calls from the medical and health informatics community have also included adding another layer of testing in addition to testing approaches those outlined earlier in this book chapter (i.e. before an AI system is deployed for real-world use) (Price and Gerke 2019). Here, physician researchers have suggested there is a need to conduct random-ized clinical control trials on AI systems before they are used to verify product claims (i.e. the quality and safety of the product being implemented is tested fully and robustly) (Price and Gerke 2019). Other researchers have suggested there is a need to conduct traditional randomized clinical control trials (i.e. the gold standard in medical research) to clearly ascertain the effects of the AI solution. For example,

Price and Gerke (2019) state that such research will be needed for medical societies to provide clear guidelines on the selection, application and use of the technology.

## 10   AI and Its Implementation

Medical and health informatics researchers have called for transparency and the development of a better understanding of algorithms and their use in specific patient and organizational contexts. Physicians are being encouraged by lawyers and professional societies to assess the value and risks associated using AI in practice and to advocate for the rigorous procurement of technologies before they are implemented in real-world settings. Some researchers have called for increased transparency from AI developers and increased physician ability to scrutinize the technology to determine its potential and actual impacts on practice (including understanding the limitations of the technology in supporting diagnostic processes and potential patient safety issues that may be introduced) (Matheny et al. 2019; Price and Gerke 2019). Price and Gerke (2019) suggest there is a need for physicians to be able to decide when and where AI is applied in their own practices (if at all). In cases where the technology is being procured by a healthcare organization, rather than a physician practice, legal scholars suggest physicians participate in vetting AI algorithms prior to engaging in procurement of such technologies (Matheny et al. 2019; Price and Gerke 2019; He et al. 2019).

## 11   Future Directions: AI and Patient Safety

AI has considerable potential to improve medical decision-making and health care processes (Matheny et al. 2019; Price and Gerke 2019; Jiang et al. 2017; He et al. 2019). Yet, as with every other health technology, it also has the potential to introduce technology-induced errors (Kushniruk et al. 2005; Koppel et al. 2005; Borycki and Kushniruk 2008; Borycki et al. 2009, 2012; Kushniruk et al. 2012; Borycki and Kushniruk 2010; Borycki et al. 2013). In our review of the literature at the intersection of AI and safety, there points to a need to undertake a comprehensive and measured research approach towards AI in its design, development, implementation and maintenance to understand its impact on patient safety. Such an approach can be drawn from employing a cognitive-socio-technical framework as outlined in Borycki and Kushniruk (2010). The approach employs the use of three differing levels to study the impacts of introducing a new technology such as AI into healthcare on patient safety (see Fig. 1).

As shown in Fig. 1, at level one, there is a need to study the impacts of AI on individual physician, health professional and administrator decision-making and reasoning processes before the technology is implemented. Here, there is a need to employ usability testing and clinical simulation approaches to understand how

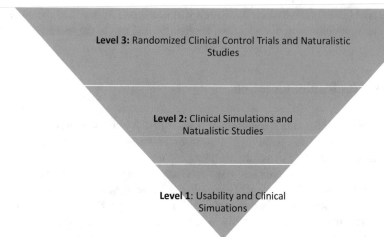

**Fig. 1** Cognitive-socio-technical framework for evaluating and researching AI—adapted from Borycki and Kushniruk (2010)

the technology affects physician decision-making and reasoning. This work would involve observing physicians' reasoning and decision-making strategies and the effects of the technology on improving physicians' decisions' as well as failing to support those decisions to better understand the limitations and boundaries of the technology in supporting work. This is important as such information is needed by physicians and researchers as well as professionals developing the technology and its guidelines for use to ensure that clinicians understand the technology's limits in supporting safe care practices as outlined above. At level two, research involving simulations and naturalistic studies could be conducted to observe how AI, when inserted into an ecosystem of other healthcare technologies performs in supporting the work of health professionals working on basic tasks. Here, there would be an opportunity to conduct clinical simulations to observe how the AI changes the way work is done in typical and atypical as well as routine and complex clinical situations and contexts. Lastly, in cases where AI supports clinical work on a healthcare systems level, such as in the case of supporting multiple users across systems, there is a need to test AI for its reproducibility in real-world contexts. Here, the technology may require some testing in settings on data sets outside the one on which it was initially developed. Validation of AI on other data sets is critical (Barber 2019). In addition to this, there is a need to recognize that investments need to be made in terms of conducting randomized clinical control trials of the technology especially in cases where it has direct impacts on human health and to provide sufficient transparency for physicians to be able to assess the technology's use in their own practice or healthcare system (Price and Gerke, 2019).

## 12   Conclusion

AI is emerging as a new and important technology that could provide significant benefits to healthcare systems (Matheny et al. 2019). Health informatics, health information technology and computer science professionals need to understand the emerging safety issues associated with introducing AI into clinical and administrative healthcare settings such as technology-induced errors, data and safety of AI solutions, safety and the role of large datasets, data safety and patient privacy and the effects of dataset quality on healthcare. Future work needs to involve the use of frameworks to evaluate AI at the individual, group and system level in order to fully understand its impacts and to identify its limitations and patient safety issues. Such an approach will be needed for improving patient safety over time as the technology matures (Borycki and Kushniruk 2010).

**Acknowledgements**  This book chapter was, in part, supported by a research grant from the Michael Smith Foundation for Health Research, British Columbia, Canada.

## References

Barber G (2019) Artificial intelligence confronts a "reproducability" crisis. Wired 2019 Sept 16, 9. https://www.wired.com/story/artificial-intelligence-confronts-reproducibility-crisis/

Bellini V, Guzzon M, Bigliardi B, Mordonini M, Filippelli S, Bignami E (2019) Artificial intelligence: a new tool in operating room management. Role of machine learning models in operating room optimization. J Med Syst 44(1):20. https://doi.org/10.1007/s10916-019-1512-1

Borycki E, Keay E (2010) Methods to assess the safety of health information systems. Healthcare quarterly (Toronto, Ont.) 13:47–52

Borycki EM, Kushniruk AW (2008) Where do technology-induced errors come from? Towards a model for conceptualizing and diagnosing errors caused by technology. In: Kushniruk AW, Borycki EM (eds) Human, Social and organizational aspects of health information systems. IGI global, Pennsylvania, pp 148–166

Borycki EM, Kushniruk AW (2010) Towards an integrative cognitive-socio-technical approach in health informatics: analyzing technology-induced error involving health information systems to improve patient safety. Open Med Inform J 15(4):181–187. https://doi.org/10.2174/187443110 1004010181

Borycki EM, Kushniruk A, Keay E, Nicoll J, Anderson J, Anderson M (2009) Toward an integrated simulation approach for predicting and preventing technology-induced errors in healthcare: implications for healthcare decision-makers. Healthc Q 12:90–96

Borycki EM, Kushniruk AW, Bellwood P, Brender J (2012) Technology-induced errors. Methods Inf Med 51(02):95–103

Borycki E, Kushniruk A, Nohr C, Takeda H, Kuwata S, Carvalho C, Bainbridge M, Kannry J (2013) Usability methods for ensuring health information technology safety: evidence-based approaches contribution of the IMIA working group health informatics for patient safety. Yearb Med Inform 8:20–7

Borycki E, Dexheimer JW, Cossio CH, Gong Y, Jensen S, Kaipio J, Kennebeck S, Kirkendall E, Kushniruk AW, Kuziemsky C, Marcilly R (2016) Methods for addressing technology-induced errors: the current state. Yearb Med Inform 25(01):30–40

Brownlee J (2019) 14 Different types of learning in machine learning. Start machine learning. https://machinelearningmastery.com/types-of-learning-in-machine-learning/

He J, Baxter SL, Xu J et al (2019) The practical implementation of artificial intelligence technologies in medicine. Nat Med 25:30–36. https://doi.org/10.1038/s41591-018-0307-0

Jiang F, Jiang Y, Zhi Y, Li H, Ma S, Wang Yl, Don Q, Shen H, Wang Y (2017) Artificial intelligence in healthcare: past, present and future. Stroke Vasular Neurol 2. https://doi.org/10.1136/svn-2017-000101

Koppel R, Metlay JP, Cohen A, Abaluck B, Localio AR, Kimmel SE, Strom BL (2005) Role of computerized physician order entry systems in facilitating medication errors. JAMA 293(10):1197–1203

Kushniruk AW, Triola MM, Borycki EM, Stein B, Kannry JL (2005) Technology induced error and usability: the relationship between usability problems and prescription errors when using a handheld application. Int J Med Inform 74(7–8):519–526. Epub 2005 Apr 8

Kushniruk A, Surich J, Borycki E (2012) Detecting and classifying technology-induced error in the transmission of healthcare data. In: 24th international conference of the European federation for medical informatics Europe 2012, 25–30 Aug 2012

Kim HE, Kim HH, Han BK, Kim KH, Han K, Nam H, Lee EH, Kim EK (2020) Changes in cancer detection and false-positive recall in mammography using artificial intelligence: a retrospective, multireader study. The Lancet Digit Health

Magrabi F, Ong MS, Runciman W, Coiera E (2012) Using FDA reports to inform a classification for health information technology safety problems. J Am Med Inform Assoc 19(1):45–53. https://doi.org/10.1136/amiajnl-2011-000369. Epub 2011 Sep 8

Menke NB, Caputo N, Fraser R, Haber J, Shields C, Menke MN (2014) A retrospective analysis of the utility of an artificial neural network to predict ED volume. Am J Emerg Med 32(6):614–617. https://doi.org/10.1016/j.ajem.2014.03.011. Epub 2014 Mar 19

Matheny ME, Whicher D, Israni ST (2019) Artificial intelligence in health care: a report from the national academy of medicine. JAMA 323(6):509–510

Palojoki S, Mäkelä M, Lehtonen L, Saranto K (2017) An analysis of electronic health record-related patient safety incidents. Health Inform J 23(2):134–145. https://doi.org/10.1177/1460458216631072. Epub 2016 Mar 7

Price WN, Gerke S (2019) Potential liability for physicians using artificial intelligence. JAMA 322(18):1765–1766

# Utilizing Health Analytics in Improving the Performance of Hospitals and Healthcare Services: Promises and Challenges

Mohamed Khalifa and Mowafa Househ

**Abstract** Health informatics is heading towards utilizing big data analytics, business intelligence, and artificial intelligence in exploring current and potential healthcare challenges and recommending evidence-based solutions to enhance strategic effectiveness and improve operational efficiency. We need to explore various advantages and potential gains of utilizing health analytics in addition to discussing different types of challenges and methods of overcoming these challenges in implementing and utilizing such resources. We conducted a focused review of literature to classify the advantages of implementing and utilizing health analytics. Health analytics challenges and critical success factors were also examined and categorised based on qualitative thematic analysis. Through examining sixty eligible studies, our focused review of literature identified three ways to classify advantages and potential gains of utilizing health analytics; based on healthcare levels, aspects, and dimensions. We also identified three main categories of challenges of health analytics: human, technological, and organisational. Using health analytics, several healthcare aspects can be improved, such as patient safety, healthcare effectiveness, efficiency, and timeliness. Health analytics implementation is faced with various technology, human, and organization related challenges. The non-technological challenges are more difficult and need more time to be resolved, including the development of a clear vision to guide implementation projects.

**Keywords** Health analytics · Big data · Business intelligence · Artificial intelligence · Healthcare performance improvement · Hospitals

M. Khalifa (✉)
Centre for Health Informatics, Australian Institute of Health Innovation, Faculty of Medicine, Health and Human Sciences, Macquarie University, Sydney, Australia
e-mail: mohamed.khalifa@mq.edu.au

M. Househ
Division of Information and Computing Technology, College of Science and Engineering, Hamad Bin Khalifa University, Qatar Foundation, Doha, Qatar

© Springer Nature Switzerland AG 2021
M. Househ et al. (eds.), *Multiple Perspectives on Artificial Intelligence in Healthcare*, Lecture Notes in Bioengineering, https://doi.org/10.1007/978-3-030-67303-1_3

# 1   Introduction

The world has experienced more than four decades of progress in digitizing health information; aggregating years of medical practice, research and development data in electronic databases. Healthcare stakeholders are now able to see new opportunities for utilizing big data, which is so called not only for its huge volume but also for its complexity, diversity, and timeliness. Health analytics supports better insights and control for making evidence-based decisions, which should help to improve quality of care and reduce costs (Groves et al. 2016). Health analytics identifies hidden values within big data. Researchers can analyse the data to explore what treatments are most effective for specific conditions or certain populations, identify patterns related to drug side effects, hospital readmissions, or emergency department waiting time (Jee and Kim 2013). Through predictive analytics, Bates et al. (2014) identified and managed common six healthcare cases, to achieve value and reduce costs. These are high-cost patients, readmissions, triage, deterioration, adverse events, and treatment optimization for diseases affecting multiple organ systems. It is reported that almost 30% of hospital readmissions in the United States are identified as avoidable, which represents a great opportunity to improve the delivered healthcare (Bates et al. 2014). A few published studies have focused on reviewing the challenges of health analytics or its benefits and opportunities (Islam et al. 2018; Kruse 2016; Mehta and Pandit 2018). However, none of these reviews discussed, in a structured and detailed approach, the different categories of challenges and the suggested approaches to overcome each category of them. In addition, these published reviews did not discuss the benefits and opportunities of health analytics applications in different healthcare services. Our study aims at exploring and reporting the advantages and potential gains of utilizing health informatics and healthcare big data analytics in addition to discussing different categories and types of challenges and the methods of overcoming these challenges in implementing and utilizing such resources.

## *1.1   Background*

In this section, we are going to present what is health analytics, what is it about, and how is it generally used to improve healthcare and clinical outcomes. In the next two sections, we are going to present some information about the functions and types of health analytics. Health analytics can be defined as a business-driven concept that includes various business intelligence approaches and big data analytics. This concept depends largely on the available and accessible data and information that are collected via well integrating and interoperable systems such as hospital information systems, electronic medical records, clinical decision support systems, and other specialized medical systems (Madsen 2012). Advanced technology applications are collecting more information than ever done. At the same time, senior leaders of healthcare organizations are eager to know whether they are getting the full value from the massive amounts of data and information they have. To know what has happened and the reason why it happened is not enough. Organizations nowadays want to know what is currently happening, what is going to happen in the future and what decisions should be made to achieve the desired outcomes (LaValle 2011). There is a logical relationship between health analytics, healthcare big data, and artificial intelligence. Big data represents the foundation on which health analytics, with its wide spectrum of technologies and methods, can work. At the same time, health analytics provides the technical and methodological framework through which artificial intelligence can be used to extract value or discover new clinical correlations out of massive health data sets (Miller and Brown 2018; Wong et al. 2019).

The Healthcare Information and Management Systems Society in the United States developed a definition for the health analytics, which includes the systematic utilization of clinical, medical, and health related data and information through implementing different analytics approaches and methodologies, such as quantitative and qualitative statistical analysis, contextual analysis, and predicting outcomes to develop decisions and actions and guide better information based strategic and operational healthcare (Cortada et al. 2012). Recently, healthcare data warehouses collect different data types from different systems and sources to create operational healthcare dashboards, strategic scorecards and data stores, since the availability of timely and accurate data is vital to make informed medical and managerial decisions (Nugawela 2013). One of the applications of big data analytics includes newly introduced approaches of employing different sources of data to predict incidents of asthma-related emergency department (ED) visits. To achieve this objective, Twitter data, Google search data, and environment data are gathered. The invented model should support predicting asthma-related ED visits using these real-time data with almost 70% accuracy. These results can be helpful for public health surveillance, ED preparedness, and targeted patient interventions (Ram 2015). Hospital based big data can also be used to design reliable predictive models and tools, which in turn can provide clinicians and decision makers with more robust and evidence-based methods for managing specific patient populations, such as cardiovascular patients (Rumsfeld et al. 2016). Recent post implementation impact studies proved that some evidence-based predictive tools, designed using big data, such as the modified early warning score, have achieved a significant reduction in the incidence of in-hospital cardiac arrests, the proportion of patients admitted to intensive care and their in-hospital mortality (Moon 2011).

## 1.2 What Does Health Analytics do?

Health analytics can help healthcare professionals and administrators to measure the performance of the various services in hospitals and healthcare organizations through establishing benchmarks to determine what is good and what is bad (Hunt 1998). There are three types of performance measures; key result indicators which should tell you how you have done, performance indicators (PIs), which should tell you what

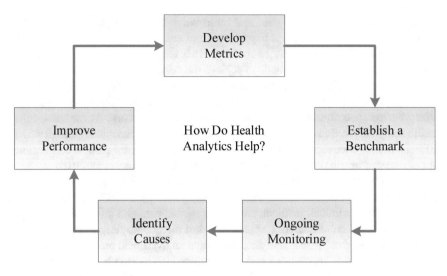

**Fig. 1** How do health analytics help improve performance?

to do and key performance indicators (KPIs), which should tell you what to do exactly to increase performance dramatically. Many performance measures used by healthcare organizations actually are an inappropriate mix of these three types (Parmenter 2015). Proper health analytics then help healthcare professionals and organizations to monitor these metrics on an ongoing and regular basis and help to troubleshoot bad performance and to identify root causes of problems. Health analytics also support users in designing, developing, implementing and evaluating diverse key performance indicators which could monitor performance, identify why performance deviation occur, and ultimately improve performance (Fisher and Analytics 2013). Figure 1 shows a simple model of how health analytics work in improving healthcare performance. Recently, many researchers are using big data analytics in developing new KPIs to reflect the actual performance of hospitals and identify methods of enhancing their healthcare efficiency. One study in Denmark used the data of over 2 million patients to develop a cost-bloom model and core KPIs related to measuring the efficiency of healthcare services provided, where a "cost bloom", is defined by the authors as "a surge in healthcare costs that propels patients from a lower to an upper decile of population-level healthcare expenditures between consecutive years" (Tamang 2017).

## *1.3   Types of Health Analytics*

The domain of health analytics is currently shifting from the lower level of operational analytics into the highest level of strategic analytics. It is also shifting

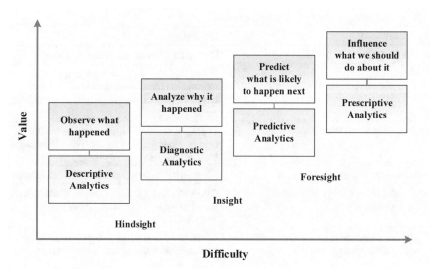

**Fig. 2** Types of health analytics

from the simplest descriptive analytics into the most complex diagnostic, predictive, and prescriptive analytics. Very soon, healthcare organizations which used descriptive and diagnostic analytics in monitoring the performance of various healthcare services, will use the most advanced types of predictive and prescriptive health analytics to choose among different feasible alternatives (Russom 2011). Figure 2 shows the four main types of health analytics discussed by most healthcare professionals and researchers and suggested by Gartner (Wang 2016).

## 2 Methods

We conducted a focused review of literature to collect and examine the reported advantages and potential gains of implementing and utilizing health analytics in improving the performance of hospitals and healthcare services. Challenges of health analytics, including reported barriers and critical success factors were also examined and categorised using qualitative thematic analysis. A comprehensive search for published evidence on "Health Analytics", "Healthcare Big Data" and "Healthcare Business Intelligence" was conducted using MEDLINE, EMBASE, CINAHL and Google Scholar for publications in available over the last ten years; from 2010 to 2020, published in English language. Table 1 shows the main keywords used in the search and their description. Figure 3 shows PRISMA flow diagram of studies selection and inclusion.

**Table 1**  Search keywords and their description

| Search keywords | Description |
|---|---|
| Health analytics | Covers all types of health data analytics |
| Healthcare big data | Managing, analyzing, or extracting health information from health data sets that are too large or complex to be dealt with by traditional methods |
| Healthcare business intelligence | Strategies and technologies used by healthcare organizations for the data analysis of healthcare business information |
| Benefits or promises or advantages | All positive outcomes of using health analytics |
| Challenges or barriers or limitations | All factors that prevent, decrease, or slow down the adoption or implementation of health analytics |
| Critical success factors or successful adoption or successful implementation | All factors that support, enhance, or facilitate successful adoption or implementation of health analytics |

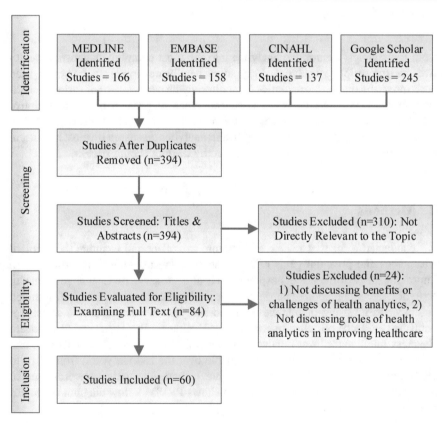

**Fig. 3**  PRISMA flow diagram of studies selection

# 3 Results

Through examining sixty eligible studies, our focused review of literature identified three ways to classify advantages and potential gains of health analytics; based on dimensions, aspects, and levels of healthcare. We also identified three main categories of challenges of health analytics: human, technology, and organization.

## 3.1 *Improving Healthcare Performance*

Improving the performance of any system depends mainly on having a shared goal that unites the interests and activities of different stakeholders. The proper goal for any healthcare delivery system is to improve the performance of services and increase the value delivered to patients (Kaplan and Porter 2011). If healthcare systems and services performance improve; patients, providers and payers will all benefit with some trade-offs in certain situations, such as the balance between increasing quality and reducing costs. Performance per se includes many of the other goals already addressed in healthcare, such as effectiveness, efficiency, quality and patient safety. It is also fundamental to achieving other important goals such as improving equity and expanding access to healthcare services at reasonable cost (Porter 2010). Healthcare stakeholders often have many goals that are naturally conflicting, such as access to services, profitability, high quality, cost containment, safety, convenience, and patient satisfaction. The Institute of Medicine's own definition of goals for the healthcare delivery system includes no less than six disparate elements: safety, effectiveness, efficiency, timeliness, patient centeredness and equity (Porter 2010). Over the years, healthcare researchers and professionals realized that many, if not all, performance dimensions are still below what is really needed or at least still have a gap that can be improved, including all the six elements defined by the Institute of Medicine. Healthcare organizations need to adopt well researched or tested procedures and technologies, well developed guidelines and standards of care, validated care protocols and multidisciplinary clinical pathways, preventing or removing unnecessary, therefore expensive, unsafe and harmful routines and procedures and reduce undesirable variations in the healthcare provision (Grol et al. 2013).

Healthcare performance improvement is facing challenges, many of them remain to be addressed, such as balancing perspectives, defining accountability, establishing criteria, identifying reporting requirements, minimizing conflict between financial and quality goals, and developing information systems (McGlynn 1997). There is a need, for example, to balance healthcare effectiveness and efficiency to gain the highest net benefit to individuals and society (Donabedian 1988). Efficiency and quality should not be mutually exclusive; the challenge is to merge economic and clinical incentives (Brook et al. 1996). The real challenge is to focus on all the important aspects of performance, using the most valid methodology possible and data evidence available, whilst trying to minimize conflicts among these competing performance aspects (Campbell et al. 2000). According to the three levels of health-care management and performance, we can classify performance measurements and their related tools, applications, and methods into operational, tactical and strategic levels. Each category has its own objectives, methods of measurement and expected outcomes (Eckerson 2009; Grigoroudis et al. 2012; Hans et al. 2012). Moreover, according to the Donabedian conceptual model, which provides a framework for evaluating healthcare services and quality of care, performance dimensions can be classified differently by being related to the three main elements of the healthcare system: structures, processes, and outcomes. Structure dimension and indicators can be used to measure and report the context through which healthcare services are delivered, including machines, buildings, people, and finance, while process dimen-sion and indicators include measuring and reporting encounters that occur between patients and healthcare professionals during the delivery of healthcare services, and outcome dimension and indicators refer to the effects of healthcare on the health status of patients and populations (Donabedian 1988; Gilbert 2015).

Using both performance levels and performance dimensions, measurable perfor-mance aspects can be classified into the main six elements defined; safety, effec-tiveness, efficiency, timeliness, patient centeredness and equity (Porter 2010; Bauer and Paradox 2014). Safety KPIs are designed to measure and report the extent at which healthcare interventions or procedures are safe and not harmful to patients or professionals. Effectiveness KPIs are designed to measure and report the extent at which healthcare service can produce the desired outcomes and fulfil the planned objectives. Efficiency KPIs are designed to measure and report the extent at which resources of healthcare organizations such as effort, time, and money are well utilized for the planned tasks and objectives. Timeliness KPIs are designed to measure and report the extent at which healthcare is delivered to patients at the most necessary or beneficial time or according to patients' understanding of need. Patient centeredness KPIs are designed to measure and report the extent at which patients are satisfied with the delivered healthcare services and the level of systems' success or failure to meet and satisfy patients' needs, including respecting patients, providing correct and accurate information, relieving patients from avoidable pain or stress. Equity KPIs are designed to measure and report the extent at which healthcare provision ensures eliminating differences between patient groups to achieve the objective of treating all patients equally and delivering best quality healthcare regardless of personal charac-teristics, such as age, gender, race, ethnicity, education, disability, sexual orientation, income, or location of residence (Brilli et al. 2014; Khalifa and Khalid 2015).

## 3.2   Challenges of Utilizing Health Analytics

It is now well-recognized that health analytics has the capacity to critically improve healthcare provision. However, the implementation of such technology is still facing different challenges. It is important to identify and define challenges to overcome and success factors to benefit from. The development and implementation of health analytics is a very complex undertaking requiring considerable resources. Yet there is a limited informative set of identified challenges and critical success factors (Yeoh and Koronios 2010). To date, little research has been done on challenges of adopting big data analytics in healthcare (Wang et al. 2015). Health analytics implementation is faced with various technology, human, and organization related challenges; examples are summarized and illustrated in Fig. 4, adapted from Khalifa, 2019 (Khalifa 2019). The non-technological challenges are more difficult and need more time to be resolved, including the development of a clear vision to guide implementation projects and achieve objectives. Successful implementation of such technology is based largely on the type of project funding, the delivered value and the alignments between project objectives and strategic organizational goals. Health analytics should be built with the end users in mind (Adamala and Cidrin 2011; Farrokhi and Pokoradi 2013). A few other studies categorized the challenges that face developing and implementing health analytics and other information systems into six main types, these include human, profession, technology, organization, funding, and regulation or legislation challenges (Khalifa 2013). Figure 5 shows the six main categories of challenges.

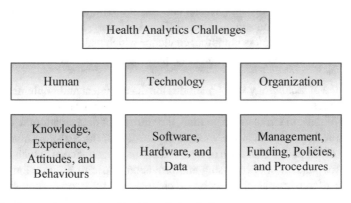

**Fig. 4** The three main categories of health analytics challenges

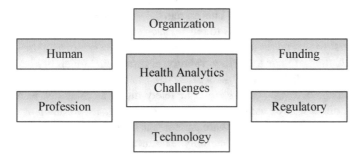

**Fig. 5** A model of six suggested categories of health analytics challenges

A few studies worked on explaining delayed or unsuccessfully implemented projects or the underutilization of health analytics technologies by linking this failure to negatively accepting or resisting these technologies by healthcare professionals. The impact of being knowledgeable, skilled, and experienced in computer systems or information technology and the attitude of healthcare professionals towards using such systems and technology in the healthcare context account for the major challenge to successfully implementing and utilizing such systems (Khalifa 2014). Other studies reported that more time and effort were needed to learn new technologies which usually resulted in longer workdays especially during the initial phase of implementing analytical or reporting systems. This might add more work, decrease productivity, or slow down performance, which can also be considered important challenges. Even highly regarded, industry-leading analytics and reporting systems can be challenging to use because of the multiplicity of functions, options and navigational tools (Khalifa 2014; Miller and Sim 2004). At the same time, health information systems research often focuses on the design and implementation challenges, but not enough focus is given to how end users react to such systems. The success of health analytics systems lies beyond the level of good design or the selection of a good system. The degree of fitting the intended use by any system leads users to accept or reject such system (Holden and Karsh 2010). The continuous need for technical and consultation support from different software, hardware, networks and other support service vendors is another challenge which makes larger hospitals more able to implement such systems because of their superior and vast resources (Lorenzi 2009).

In the area of technology which includes the development and implementation of health analytics, we might be able to identify many challenges in relation to the huge expansion of data, in terms of the volume, the velocity of data creation, which might be even more important than the volume, especially for the real-time analysis, and the variety of big data, in the form of text, voice, images and videos, which is another challenge for acquisition, processing and provision of useful information (McAfee et al. 2012). Moreover, one of the technical challenges is the trade-off between generalisability and customisation of health analytics solutions. Some of these solutions are developed using local data. For example, some predictive models were developed using life quality, expectancy scores, or national rates of diseases from certain populations in specific countries. This affects the willingness of patients, clinicians, and other healthcare professionals to rely on such solutions in decision making. It is also essential sometimes to make major adjustments to the health analytics solutions and re-evaluation of their feasibility, validity, accuracy, and reliability before using them in other populations (Khalifa et al. 2019). In addition to the technical aspects of data management we still have a completely different challenge in relation to the ethical dimension of using and sharing patient data. How clinicians and other healthcare professionals use and share patient data should always include protecting patients' privacy and data confidentiality. The increased use of big data analytics and artificial intelligence methods requires reassessment of these basic principles and available legislations, regulations, policies, and procedures, while managing the emerging concerns of patients privacy, data confidentiality, data ownership, and informed patients' consent on using and sharing their data. Accordingly, different stakeholders must have conversations about the appropriate approaches to manage these issues and support the development of such capability in the most just, ethical manner possible (Balthazar 2018).

Yet, developing and implementing health analytics is not only about introducing new technology, this is more about equipping healthcare organizations by tools that enable them to achieve their healthcare objectives and providing users with technical capabilities that make new things possible and by engaging people into changing their behaviours to effectively use the new capabilities to achieve the target outcomes. Top level management commitment and developing policies and procedures governing the implementation and utilization of applications is another crucial organizational challenge (McCarthy and Eastman 2013). Some studies discussed managerial challenges facing the utilization of big data and analytics. Healthcare senior management that assigns smart objectives, develops standards of success, and looks for the right answers is even more important than developing only bigger data; the necessity of a human understanding and insights cannot be simply replaced by powerful analytics. Talent management is another challenge, since data content become cheaper, human input becomes more valuable. The challenge of selecting the right tools to manage big data is another managerial issue. The successful effective evidence-based decision making is another challenge for the management in addition to changing the organization culture from "what we think" to "what we know" (McAfee et al. 2012); identifying organizational top level management information needs (Trkman 2010). Moreover, the increased initial costs, operational and maintenance costs, and uncertain financial benefits of health information systems are frequently cited barriers to the acquisition and implementation of such systems. In addition, some concerns might be raised in the form of ethical and legal questions about the proper acquisition and utilization of systems. Health information confidentiality is one of these factors (Kellermann and Jones 2013).

All these challenges can be classified into three major classes: technological, human, and organizational. They can also be interrelated and interdependent since the development and implementation of information systems is a process of mutual transformation. The organization, the technology and the human behaviours could transform each other during these processes; one way would be to look at behavioural influences on health analytics outcomes in the context of institutional constraints. When this is expected, the process of acquiring and implementing a new system can be planned strategically to help accomplishing the transformation of the healthcare organization. This major change project can succeed only when positively and effectively supported by both top level management and future users (Berg 2001). Published research discusses that technology related factors, such as hardware, software, and data content, is more influential on the descriptive function of analytics rather than on the prescriptive function. On the other hand, human related factors, such as knowledge, experience and skills can be more influential on the prescriptive analytics rather than on the descriptive. The domain of analytics and big data is faced mainly by two challenges: (1) the engineering and technology challenge; this includes the efficient management of large data sets, and (2) the semantics of human knowledge and experience challenge; this includes the ability to find and meaningfully combine information that is relevant to our concern (Bizer 2012). Data volume, velocity, streaming, aggregation, and data variety represent a major challenge facing data processing and visualization for proper descriptive and predictive analytics (Keim 2008). Many hardware and software design challenges might largely influence descriptive and predictive functions of analytics. The design of systems and components that work effectively for health analytics to generate accurate data descriptions and informative predictive models requires an understanding of both the needs of users and the technologies used. Developers must design good interfaces, easy to understand graphics, and easy to use icons to improve the organization of applications and their related functionalities. Other technology related challenges might include data quality versus quantity, data growth and expansion, system speed and system scale, unstructured data, data compliance, security and distributed processing (Kaisler, et al. 2013). As health analytics is one of the most recently introduced technologies, it requires the contribution and innovation of professionals with the highest levels of training, knowledge, and experience, in addition to many other essential skills. These skills must include the ability to conduct research, critical analysis, and creativity, in order to enhance using prescriptive analytics and advising organizations on possible outcomes and answer the question of what should we do next (Evans and Lindner 2012; Katal et al. 2013). Organizational leadership, managerial styles and some other administrative and legal related factors, such as financial issues, policies and procedures play an important role as mediating factors for other technology and human factors (LaValle 2011; Chen et al. 2012).

If the organizations are not ready yet for this kind of change, in relation to the culture and responsiveness, then diverse technology and human investments would not be sufficient to support this kind of transformation (Watson and Wixom 2007). Some studies associate different types of challenges to different levels of analytics. Data quality and readiness is an important determinant of successful operational analytics. IT infrastructure, hardware and software help a lot in building valid and accurate operational models and providing daily support for operational managers (Taylor 2010). On the other hand, tactical and more importantly strategic analytics need higher user skills and experience in extracting meaning and value from data after visualization and description. The input of human knowledge and experience into strategic analytics is more challenging, important and influential than into operational analytics, which can be more data driven than knowledge or experience driven, where strategic organizational intelligence results from, but more important than, individual transformation (Davenport 2009; Liebowitz 2006).

## 4 Discussion

Health analytics can be used on variable levels, mainly on the individual level of clinicians and healthcare professionals, on the level of hospitals and healthcare provider organizations as well as on the level of healthcare government organizations.

## 4.1 Clinicians and Healthcare Professionals

Clinicians should have the access to utilise health analytics on the levels of individual patients as well as on the public health level. On the patient level, health analytics can help CDS, evidence-based medicine and personalised medicine. Predictive analytics tools developed and validated using millions of patient records are now used more routinely by clinicians in predicting deterioration of patients in the intensive care, the need for special resources in the ER, readmission or mortality risk (Charlson 1987; Schonfeld et al. 2014; Walraven 2010). On the public health, clinicians are also be interested to use health analytics to predict resource utilisation of their services and how to improve clinical effectiveness and patient safety during their specialised care provision (Rumsfeld et al. 2016).

## 4.2 Hospitals, Insurance, Pharmaceutical and Other Companies

Hospitals, health insurance in addition to other pharmaceutical and healthcare companies are perfect candidates for using health analytics in improving their businesses. Hospitals can use predictive analytics to better prepare for the changing or increasing demand of their services after an outbreak, a seasonal variation pattern or a natural disaster (Raghupathi and Raghupathi 2014). Some newly introduced tools developed by professionals and scientists, for the analysis of healthcare insurance claims, shows how big data can support detecting fraud, abuse, and errors. Claim anomalies detected using these applications help private health insurers identify hidden cost overruns that transaction processing systems can't detect (Srinivasan and Arunasalam 2013). Pharmaceutical companies can also benefit from health analytics. By tracking which physicians prescribe which drugs and for what purposes, companies can decide whom to target, show what is the least expensive or most effective treatment plan for a disease, help identify physicians whose practices are suited to specific clinical trials (treating a large number of a specific group of patients), and map the course of an epidemic to support pharmaceutical salespersons, physicians, and patients (Koh and Tan 2011). Other healthcare services and biomedical product companies can benefit as well from the applications of big data health analytics through better understanding of the markets, patients' needs and critical success factors of biomedical devices and other products, so that they can inform their research and refine their strategies (Bollier et al. 2010).

## *4.3   Healthcare Government Organizations*

The ministry of health and other government agencies are more interested in providing better health to the people while cost-effectively utilizing available resources. The government can utilise distinct types of health analytics to enhance the value of healthcare provided to people through analyzing the needs for services, geographical distribution of such needs and demands on levels of services (Heitmueller 2014; Parikh et al. 2016; Wang et al. 2016). Improving healthcare accessibility, cost-effectiveness, and equity are among the top priorities of the Australian government (Carter 2008). Governments of many leading countries, including Australia, United States, United Kingdom and Japan, started implementing big data analytics, mainly predictive health analytics, to enhance the control and responsiveness of the government healthcare system to the changing population needs (Kim et al. 2014).

## 5   Conclusions

Today we are shifting from the lower level of operational analytics into the higher level of strategic analytics and from simple descriptive analytics toward more sophisticated diagnostic, predictive and prescriptive health analytics. Using big data and health analytics, several healthcare performance aspects can be improved, such as patient safety, healthcare effectiveness, efficiency, and timeliness. Health analytics implementation is faced with various technology, human, and organization related challenges. The non-technological challenges are more difficult and need more time to be resolved, including the development of a clear vision to guide implementation projects and achieve objectives. Some studies associate different types of challenges to different levels of analytics. Technical factors, including software, hardware and data quality are important determinants of successful operational analytics. On the other hand, tactical and more importantly strategic analytics might need higher user skills and experience in extracting meaning and value from data after visualization and description. Health analytics can be used on variable levels, mainly on the individual level of clinicians and healthcare professionals, on the level of hospitals and healthcare provider organizations as well as on the level of healthcare government organizations.

Among the main future research directions is addressing some important research gaps in the areas of developing, implementing, and utilizing health analytics in supporting and improving the provision of healthcare services. More research is needed to suggest detailed and specific plans to overcome different types of barriers and challenges of developing, implementing, and utilizing health analytics. The suggested research should investigate methods of overcoming technological, human, and organisational challenges. It should also discuss approaches to identify and prioritise such challenges, so that each healthcare organisation can work on their own priorities and target their most resistant challenges.

# References

Adamala S, Cidrin L (2011) Key success factors in business intelligence

Balthazar P et al (2018) Protecting your patients' interests in the era of big data, artificial intelligence, and predictive analytics. J Am Coll Radiol 15(3):580–586

Bates DW et al (2014) Big data in health care: using analytics to identify and manage high-risk and high-cost patients. Health Aff 33(7):1123–1131

Bauer JC (2014) Paradox and imperatives in health care: redirecting reform for efficiency and effectiveness. CRC Press

Berg M (2001) Implementing information systems in health care organizations: myths and challenges. Int J Med Inform 64(2):143–156

Bizer C et al (2012) The meaningful use of big data: four perspectives–four challenges. ACM SIGMOD Rec 40(4):56–60

Bollier D, Firestone CM (2010) The promise and peril of big data. Aspen Institute Communications and Society Program, Washington, DC

Brilli RJ, Allen S, Davis JT (2014) Revisiting the quality chasm. Pediatrics 133(5):763–765

Brook RH, McGlynn EA, Cleary PD (1996) Measuring quality of care. Mass Medical Soc

Campbell SM, Roland MO, Buetow SA (2000) Defining quality of care. Soc Sci Med 51(11):1611–1625

Carter R et al (2008) Priority setting in health: origins, description and application of the Australian assessing cost-effectiveness initiative. Expert Rev Pharmacoecon Outcomes Res 8(6):593–617

Charlson ME et al (1987) A new method of classifying prognostic comorbidity in longitudinal studies: development and validation. J Chronic Dis 40(5):373–383

Chen H, Chiang RH, Storey VC (2012) Business intelligence and analytics: from big data to big impact. MIS Q 36(4)

Cortada JW, Gordon D, Lenihan B (2012) The value of analytics in healthcare. IBM Institute for Business Value IBM, Global Business Service

Davenport TH (2009) The Rise of Strategic Analytics. AnalyticsMagazine.com. http://analytics.inf orms.org

Donabedian A (1988) The quality of care: how can it be assessed? JAMA 260(12):1743–1748

Eckerson WW (2009) Performance management strategies. Bus Intell J 14(1):24–27

Evans JR, Lindner CH (2012) Business analytics: the next frontier for decision sciences. Decis Line 43(2):4–6

Farrokhi V, Pokoradi L (2013) Organizational and technical factors for implementing business intelligence. Fascicle Manage Technol Eng 75–78

Fisher NI (2013) Analytics for leaders: a performance measurement system for business success. Cambridge University Press.

Gilbert SM (2015) Revisiting structure, process, and outcome. Cancer 121(3):328–330

Grigoroudis E, Orfanoudaki E, Zopounidis C (2012) Strategic performance measurement in a healthcare organisation: a multiple criteria approach based on balanced scorecard. Omega 40(1):104–119

Grol R et al (2013) Improving patient care: the implementation of change in health care. Wiley

Groves P et al (2016) The 'big data' revolution in healthcare: accelerating value and innovation

Hans EW, Van Houdenhoven M, Hulshof PJ (2012) A framework for healthcare planning and control. Handbook of healthcare system scheduling. Springer, pp 303–320

Heitmueller A et al (2014) Developing public policy to advance the use of big data in health care. Health Aff 33(9):1523–1530

Holden RJ, Karsh B-T (2010) The technology acceptance model: its past and its future in health care. J Biomed Inform 43(1):159–172

Hunt DL et al (1998) Effects of computer-based clinical decision support systems on physician performance and patient outcomes: a systematic review. JAMA 280(15):1339–1346

Islam MS et al (2018) A systematic review on healthcare analytics: application and theoretical perspective of data mining. Healthcare. Multidisciplinary Digital Publishing Institute.

Jee K, Kim G-H (2013) Potentiality of big data in the medical sector: focus on how to reshape the healthcare system. Healthc Inform Res 19(2):79–85

Kaisler S et al (2013) Big data: issues and challenges moving forward. In: 2013 46th Hawaii international conference on system sciences (HICSS). IEEE

Kaplan RS, Porter ME (2011) How to solve the cost crisis in health care. Harv Bus Rev 89(9):46–52

Katal A, Wazid M, Goudar R (2013) Big data: issues, challenges, tools and good practices. In: 2013 Sixth International Conference on Contemporary Computing (IC3). IEEE

Keim D et al (2008) Visual analytics: definition, process, and challenges. Lect Notes Comput Sci 4950:154–176

Kellermann AL, Jones SS (2013) What it will take to achieve the as-yet-unfulfilled promises of health information technology. Health Aff 32(1):63–68

Khalifa M (2013) Barriers to health information systems and electronic medical records implementation. A field study of Saudi Arabian hospitals. Procedia Comput Sci 21:335–342

Khalifa M (2014) Technical and human challenges of implementing hospital information systems in Saudi Arabia. J Health Inform Developing Countries 8(1)

Khalifa M (2019) Challenges of health analytics utilization: a review of literature. In: ICIMTH

Khalifa M, Khalid P (2015) Developing strategic health care key performance indicators: a case study on a tertiary care hospital. Procedia Comput Sci 63:459–466

Khalifa M, Magrabi F, Gallego B (2019) Developing a framework for evidence-based grading and assessment of predictive tools for clinical decision support. BMC Med Inform Decis Mak 19(1):207

Kim G-H, Trimi S, Chung J-H (2014) Big-data applications in the government sector. Commun ACM 57(3):78–85

Koh HC, Tan G (2011) Data mining applications in healthcare. J Healthc Inf Manage 19(2):65

Kruse CS et al (2016) Challenges and opportunities of big data in health care: a systematic review. JMIR Med Inform 4(4):e38

LaValle S et al (2011) Big data, analytics and the path from insights to value. MIT Sloan Manag Rev 52(2):21

Liebowitz J (2006) Strategic intelligence: business intelligence, competitive intelligence, and knowledge management. CRC Press

Lorenzi NM et al (2009) How to successfully select and implement electronic health records (EHR) in small ambulatory practice settings. BMC Med Inform Decis Mak 9(1):15

Madsen L (2012) Healthcare business intelligence: a guide to empowering successful data reporting and analytics. Wiley

McAfee A, Brynjolfsson E, Davenport TH (2012) Big data: the management revolution. Harv Bus Rev 90(10):60–68

McCarthy C, Eastman D (2013) Change management strategies for an effective EMR implementation. Himss

McGlynn EA (1997) Six challenges in measuring the quality of health care. Health Aff 16(3):7–21

Mehta N, Pandit A (2018) Concurrence of big data analytics and healthcare: a systematic review. Int J Med Inform 114:57–65

Miller DD, Brown EW (2018) Artificial intelligence in medical practice: the question to the answer? Am J Med 131(2):129–133

Miller RH, Sim I (2004) Physicians' use of electronic medical records: barriers and solutions. Health Aff 23(2):116–126

Moon A et al (2011) An eight year audit before and after the introduction of modified early warning score (MEWS) charts, of patients admitted to a tertiary referral intensive care unit after CPR. Resuscitation 82(2):150–154

Nugawela S (2013) Data warehousing model for integrating fragmented electronic health records from disparate and heterogeneous clinical data stores. Queensland University of Technology.

Parikh RB, Kakad M, Bates DW (2016) Integrating predictive analytics into high-value care: the dawn of precision delivery. JAMA 315(7):651–652

Parmenter D (2015) Key performance indicators: developing, implementing, and using winning KPIs. Wiley

Porter ME (2010) What is value in health care? N Engl J Med 363(26):2477–2481

Raghupathi W, Raghupathi V (2014) Big data analytics in healthcare: promise and potential. Health Inf Sci Syst 2(1):3

Ram S et al (2015) Predicting asthma-related emergency department visits using big data. IEEE J Biomed Health Inform 19(4):1216–1223

Rumsfeld JS, Joynt KE, Maddox TM (2016) Big data analytics to improve cardiovascular care: promise and challenges. Nat Rev Cardiol 13(6):350–359

Russom P (2011) Big data analytics. TDWI Best Practices Report, Fourth Quarter 19:40

Schonfeld D et al (2014) Pediatric emergency care applied research network head injury clinical prediction rules are reliable in practice. Archives of disease in childhood archdischild-2013–305004

Srinivasan U, Arunasalam B (2013) Leveraging big data analytics to reduce healthcare costs. IT Prof 15(6):21–28

Tamang S et al (2017) Predicting patient 'cost blooms' in Denmark: a longitudinal population-based study. BMJ Open 7(1):e011580

Taylor J (2010) Operational analytics: putting analytics to work in operational systems. BeyeNetwork

Trkman P (2010) The critical success factors of business process management. Int J Inf Manage 30(2):125–134

van Walraven C et al (2010) Derivation and validation of an index to predict early death or unplanned readmission after discharge from hospital to the community. Can Med Assoc J 182(6):551–557

Wang Y et al (2015) Beyond a technical perspective: understanding big data capabilities in health care. In: 2015 48th Hawaii international conference on system sciences (HICSS). IEEE

Wang FF (2016) Healthcare information analytic

Wang Y, Kung L, Byrd TA (2016) Big data analytics: Understanding its capabilities and potential benefits for healthcare organizations. Technol Forecast Soc Chang

Watson HJ, Wixom BH (2007) The current state of business intelligence. Computer 40(9)

Wong ZS, Zhou J, Zhang Q (2019) Artificial intelligence for infectious disease big data analytics. Infect Dis Health 24(1):44–48

Yeoh W, Koronios A (2010) Critical success factors for business intelligence systems. J Comput Inf Syst 50(3):23–32

# Perspectives on Human-AI Interaction Applied to Health and Wellness Management: Between Milestones and Hurdles

**Mohammed Tahri Sqalli, Dena Al-Thani, Marwa Qaraqe, and Luis Fernandez-Luque**

**Abstract** Across the globe, the demand over a good quality healthcare is in the rise. Patients require rigorous treatments and thorough followups. Meanwhile, the advent of artificial intelligence has opened up various opportunities for healthcare providers to meet their patients' demands. With the use of artificial intelligence, data can be harnessed to provide digital guidance, design care management programs, as well as predict the upcoming health crisis. While artificial intelligence for managing patients' health and well-being may seem ready to be implemented, patients as well as health institutions still devote a preponderant importance to the clinician at the center of care. In this chapter, we explore the position of artificial intelligence in the management of health and well-being, where the human (patient) to human (clinician) interaction is key to its success. Yet, patients feel ready to get support from artificial intelligence. We first describe opportunities of how artificial intelligence is already used in the management of patients' health. We then describe the hurdles impeding the Human-AI interaction between the artificial intelligent health management systems and the user.

**Keywords** Human-AI interaction · Machine learning · Digital medicine · Health informatics

M. T. Sqalli (✉) · D. Al-Thani · M. Qaraqe · L. Fernandez-Luque
Hamad Bin Khalifa University, Qatar Foundation Division of Information Computing Technology
College of Science and Engineering, Doha, Qatar
e-mail: mtahrisqalli@hbku.edu.qa

D. Al-Thani
e-mail: dalthani@hbku.edu.qa

M. Qaraqe
e-mail: mqaraqe@hbku.edu.qa

L. Fernandez-Luque
e-mail: lluque@hbku.edu.qa

© Springer Nature Switzerland AG 2021
M. Househ et al. (eds.), *Multiple Perspectives on Artificial Intelligence in Healthcare*,
Lecture Notes in Bioengineering, https://doi.org/10.1007/978-3-030-67303-1_4

# 1 Introduction

The advancements in hardware as well as in machine learning (ML) have diversified the fields of application for artificial intelligence (AI) systems. Among the applications of these systems are in the medical field. This progress brought techniques for processing vast amounts of patients' generated data into several modalities. It has also allowed the conversion of multiple data streams collected by ubiquitous computing devices into unified feedback models. These models provide medical emergency insights, timely medical reminders, as well as accurate medical predictions (Koh and Tan 2005; Sqalli and Al-Thani 2019). The drive for improving medical interventions has thus pushed the movement of digitalizing health institutions through the adoption of these intelligent systems. AI systems are now a tool for supplementing clinicians' decision making, for providing customized and tailored health management plans, for predicting the next health crisis, and for designing personalized treatments using precision medicine (Chancellor et al. 2016).

However, with the prevalent adoption of machine learning into the medical context, these AI systems have also drawn attention to the social challenges they bring. These challenges range from how classification algorithms show bias or disadvantage a certain population group over another, or how the black-box aspect of these algorithms makes them difficult to be supervised by clinicians (Inkpen et al. 2019). Moreover, AI systems have also brought concerns among the research and medical community with regards to issues of discrimination, fairness and accountability (Koh and Tan 2005; Inkpen et al. 2019). To address these issues, machine learning engineers have emphasized on proposing mathematical insights to correct these social biases, and to improve the interpretability of the classifications algorithms (Dwork et al. 2012). This field of research by itself has witnessed an exponential growth in the past decade, as it is proven by several academic venues that address such topics. These venues include but are not limited to the ACM Fairness, Accountability, and Transparency (FAT*) conferences (Proceedings of the Conference on Fairness 2019; Inkpen et al. 2019), and other related workshops. Moreover, two of the United Nations (UN) agencies, mainly the Wolrd Health Orgamization (WHO) and the International Communication Unit (ITU), have pointed out the urgency of addressing those topics by establishing a focus group dedicated for Artificial Intelligence for Health (AI4H) in July, 2018 (Wiegand et al. 2019). Among the main goals of this group is to set the regulations for evaluating and benchmarking the ethics of forthcoming AI systems for health (Wiegand et al. 2019). Allowing these topics to be discussed sets the ground for an accountable and ethical deployment of artificial intelligence in the medical context.

In the health and wellness domain, a responsible deployment of artificial intelligence using mathematical insights for biases correction is not enough (Inkpen et al. 2019). The human responsibility is still critical, if not primary. In this context, artificial intelligence and machine learning systems serve as a helping tool or as an extension to the clinician decision making process (Inkpen et al. 2019). While these systems provide accurate predictions and insights, the final say goes back to the clinician who asses the indicators provided. Based on these indicators and other medical factors, the decision taken is the one that is foreseen to be the best for the well being of the patient.

Despite their accuracy, several machine learning systems suffer from being developed by engineers in isolation and without the inclusion of clinicians and patients (Inkpen et al. 2019). The human involvement in AI systems' conception, design, development and evaluation is essential to guarantee that the insights provided by these systems are meaningful, significant and actionable for clinicians. Moreover, these systems need to be developed in an understandable and context-aware manner for the medical community. The Human-AI interaction sub-field of Human-Computer Interaction focuses on these issues. Nevertheless, it still is unclear how future emerging trends of a swiftly developing AI may lead. Due to the novelty of the field, the human-AI interaction in the medical context is still emerging, especially with regards to technologies of decision support or expert systems being deployed and tested in-the-wild (Inkpen et al. 2019).

Moreover, it is essential to prevent unintended repercussions that these expert medical systems cause. The consequences vary between biases, data interpretation errors, privacy issues, accountability, loss of trust by medical practitioners, and irresponsible usage (Lazer et al. 2014). In addition, the decision-making process in the medical setting is subjective and contextual depending on a patient case by case basis. These two aspects of specificity are challenging to account for with the standard workflow of current machine learning models. Thus, there is an imminent need for artificial intelligence systems that account for sustainable, interactive, usable, context-aware and actionable features that lead towards an integrated human-AI interaction (Inkpen et al. 2019). The involvement of the patient or clinician in this ecosystem requires a human-centered approach, where the insights provided by these decision support systems are contextual. Enabling a context-aware AI model requires accounting for the different users' differences, demands, cultural contexts, aspirations and preferences (Olteanu et al. 2019).

The goal of this chapter is to investigate at what extent the human-AI interaction is being brought to the foreground during the design, development, and use of artificial intelligent systems in the management of health and wellness. Not much research has addressed this area of interest. This chapter is founded on the novel work of Amershi et al. (2019) proposing guidelines for incorporating Human-AI interaction in the design of health and wellness solutions. This work is the first to provide a multi-perspective analysis on how to use the guidelines of human-AI interaction proposed by Amershi et al. (2019) in the health and wellness management. This chapter is structured as followed. In the next two sections, we explain respectively the milestones crossed, as well as the hurdles impeding the human-AI interaction in the health and wellness. Table 1 summarizes these milestones achieved as well as the hurdles challenging the Human-AI Interaction between the patients and the AI systems that support them in managing their health and wellness.

**Table 1** Milestones achieved and hurdles challenging the human-AI interaction in the management of patients' health and wellness

| Milestones achieved | Challenging hurdles |
|---|---|
| **1. Understandable, and explainable AI**: Artificial intelligence is currently more understandable and explainable. It is now commercialized and democratized. It is also accessible for both clinicians and patients as a secondary diagnostic tool | **1. Artificial Intelligence Literacy**: The artificial intelligence literacy among clinicians is very limited, which prohibits their involvement in the design and building of machine learning systems adequate for the clinical setting |
| **2. Documentation as an Integral Part of the Development Process**: With the understandabilty of artificial intelligence in health and wellness management, providing documentation to the machine learning tools has witnessed a progressive leap | **2. Opaque Nature of Machine Learning Algorithms**: The black-box aspect of the inner neural network layers of a machine learning model is also a barrier to understandability among clinicians |
| **3. Incorporating Both Artificial Intelligence and Human Intelligence**: In the health and wellness sector, clinicians are still at the center of care. However, artificial intelligence is being used as a helping diagnostic tool | **3. The Design over Data versus Data over Design Paradigm Dilemma**: Accounting for an effective Human-AI interaction requires to consider the design of this interaction first before the nature of the data required. However, the training process in machine learning requires the opposite. This paradigm trade-off is a nuisance to an effective Human-AI interaction |
| **4. The Birth of Human-AI Interaction**: The digitalization of health institutions has directed the attention from human-computer interaction as a general field to the introduction of Human-AI interaction for health and wellness applications as a sub-field | **4. Control of Customized Functionalities for Niche User Segments**: There is a shift towards providing a customized interface design for each user of the medical system. Classical HCI evaluation metrics do not account for the multiplicity and fluidity of interfaces depending on each individual user |
| | **5. Foreseeing the unforeseeable—Adapting to an Ever Changing Human-AI Interaction**: Both the field of medicine and machine learning algorithm design are constantly evolving. So is the interaction between the clinician and the AI system. Foreseeing these changes and expecting them is both challenging and critical to maintain a meaningful human-AI interaction |

## 2 Milestones

We list four milestones achieved in putting forward the human at the center of the human-AI interaction process.

## 2.1 Understandable, and Explainable AI

Artificial intelligence technology is now commercialized and democratized for the average user. Patients nowadays rely on AI-infused applications to manage their chronic conditions and monitor their health and wellness (Sqalli and Al-Thani 2019). Human-AI interaction experts crossed a milestone to transform AI from a deeply complex tool to a familiar and user-friendly one. Patients as well as clinicians are able to both effectively understand and explain the insights provided by the AI systems (2019). Human-AI interaction experts have also succeeded in bridging the chasm between the complexity of the neural networks for machine learning models and the simplicity of the interface enabling the patients and clinicians to easily use these AI capabilities (Adadi and Berrada, 2018).

## 2.2 Documentation as an Integral Part of the Development Process

Documentation in the medical field is of crucial importance for the safety of patients. It is the key to delivering the best error free care possible (Amira et al. 2019). Artificial intelligence for healthcare has also adopted that same mantra in order to meet the rigorous needs of the medical sector. Machine learning as well as HCI experts realize the importance of understanding how models and datasets are more usable when they are properly documented (Proceedings of the Conference on Fairness 2019). Moreover, health practitioners on the ground are advocating medical routines leading to well-documented datasets (Piwek et al. 2016; Inkpen et al. 2019).

## 2.3 Incorporating both Artificial Intelligence and Human Intelligence

The capabilities that both human intelligence and artificial intelligence offer are complementary to accomplish complex analytical tasks. While machine learning systems are effective tools to distill vast amounts of data into insights and patterns that might be invisible to clinicians. Human intelligence is effective at drawing meaningful context-relevant inferences from those patterns (Inkpen et al. 2019). Among the application of this fundamental idea is the combination of machine learning techniques along with multiscale modeling (Alber et al. 2019). Moreover, another example of the application of this concept is the use of augmented reality to initiate and improve the learning for children and adolescents with autism spectrum disorder Khowaja et al. (2020). This combination provides even more accurate predictive models. These models lead to uncovering insights about disease mechanisms, treatment strategies, and clinical decision making (Alber et al. 2019). Human-AI interaction therefore has crossed the milestone of setting the research design problems that are most suitable and are most relevant to the clinical context. Allowing both artificial intelligence and human intelligence to work in synergy guarantees the delivery of a more precise care management plan (Sqalli and Al-Thani 2019; Inkpen et al. 2019).

## 2.4  The Birth of Human-AI Interaction

The involvement of artificial intelligence in the field of human computer interaction has given birth to the human-AI interaction as a sub-field (Dove et al. 2017). The clinical setting is more and more referring to powerful machine learning algorithms, along with HCI tools to find solutions to complex diseases like cancer, genetic problems and heart problems (Turakhia et al. 2019). ML tools and HCI tools are essential in order to design analytical solutions tailored to the needs of health and wellness management (Dove et al. 2017). Both of these tools are used under the light of a translational perspective to contribute towards clinical development (Shah et al. 2019). This perspective of AI/ML—HCI has resulted in some successful outcomes in the field of cardiology (Turakhia et al. 2019), pattern recognition and segmentation techniques on medical images (Shah et al. 2019), tele-robitics care for the elderly (Sqalli et al. 2016), remote control for surgeries (Kurabe et al. 2016; Yamashita et al. 2016), and most generally health lifestyle data-driven applications using pervasive computing (Fernandez-Luque et al. 2019) among other applications.

## 3  Hurdles

We list five hurdles that challenge putting forward the human at the center of the human-AI interaction process.

## 3.1  Artificial Intelligence Literacy

The medical community suffers from artificial intelligence illiteracy (Dove et al. 2017; Yang et al. 2018). Although AI systems are progressively intruding the medical field, many patients and clinicians are still hesitant to involve those systems in their workflow (Inkpen et al. 2019; Yang et al. 2018). Dove et al. (2017) have explained how AI is currently viewed as "a magic wand" by clinicians due to their limited literacy. Lack of understanding of the current possibilities and limitations of artificial intelligence causes health practitioner users to have over-ambitions expectations from these system and algorithms (Dove et al. 2017). Limited literacy of AI therefore obscures the human integration that the field of HCI adopts. However, despite their limited AI literacy, clinicians use medical software systems that embed an aspect of AI in them (Amershi et al. 2019). Automated ECG interpretations (Turakhia et al. 2019), vital signs monitoring Piwek et al. (2016), and tele-medicine applications (Marvel et al. 2018) and others embed an important portion of artificial intelligence in them. Other health practitioners have blindly adopted those systems without much knowledge about their capabilities and inner functioning. Having little literacy about a certain technology does not prohibit using it under the premise that the clinician would use it cautiously. Human-AI interaction as a sub-field of HCI faces the challenge of designing intuitively those medical systems with the end-user, either as a patient or as a clinician, being uninvolved. Accounting for the end user when designing those systems breaks the barrier of illiteracy.

## 3.2 Opaque Nature of Machine Learning Algorithms

The black-box aspect of machine learning algorithms is another hurdle that impedes involving health practitioners in the design of medical systems. This is due mainly to a shift from an open-source software mentality to the ideology of privatization of data adopted by tech giants (Wilbanks and Topol 2016). The opaque nature of neural networks makes the task of dissecting the rules leading to the final model output difficult for clinicians. While in knowledge-based artificial intelligent systems data is represented in an understandable if-then rule knowledge-base, in neural networks, data is represented across a complex network. This representation makes the interpretability of the output impossible by novices (Adadi and Berrada, 2018). Moreover, potential anomalies hidden in the training data may cause biased or wrong output decisions (Pedreschi et al. 2019). Designing a medical-tailored machine learning model from the ground-up demands a participatory design approach. In this approach, both clinical expertise as well as the curation of a tailored machine learning model is required. By adopting this design approach, there is a potential for minimizing the biases and wrong medical interpretations. This leads to the conception of several AI development frameworks, whereby a plethora of algorithms, paradigms, as well as documentations stating the pros and cons of each framework are made available (Pedreschi et al. 2019). However, some of these frameworks according to Gillies et al. (2016) lack the transparency required for clinicians to understand the inner functioning of the algorithms. Moreover, adopting an existing AI development framework entails adopting its biases and flaws. This shapes how health practitioners interact with these systems. It also redirects their attention from the patient to addressing the biases of the used system (Pedreschi et al. 2019).

### 3.3 The Design over Data Versus Data over Design Paradigm Dilemma

Designing for an effective Human-AI interaction in the health domain stands at a crossroads between setting the priorities of the design process and the data analysis process. In the HCI human-centered design paradigm, designers aim to deduce insights and elucidate requirements for user needs (Fogg 2002; Norman 2002) before starting data collection, while in the data-centered design paradigm data scientists give the priority to the data. This creates tension with the design-first approach. The tension culminates when there is a need for identifying the pieces of data that are appropriate to the medical problem without any prior involvement of the end user. This tension leads to demanding more time for the design process, which then results in requiring more development time and more budget allocation (Yang et al. 2018). On the other end of the spectrum, in the data-centered design paradigm, machine learning models are trained using medical data that is already available, but without any specifications about the usefulness of the output for the clinician. This leads to an increase in the chances that the the output of the machine learning systems not fit the medical problem specifications.

### 3.4 Control over Customized Functionalities for Niche User Segments

Artificial intelligence has enabled the creation of customized sub-functionalities and behavior change modules within AI-infused health applications and platforms (Sqalli and Al-Thani 2019). Designers find the task of controlling the design workflow of each customized feature challenging (Inkpen et al. 2019). This abundance of features and functionalities creates a point of tension for Human-AI interaction experts. Personalized trends derived from patient data is becoming mainstream. Moreover, there is a potential that this personalization process will extend to be reflected on the design of the interface of those applications as well (Sqalli and Al-Thani 2019). Machine learning algorithms hold a potential to design drastically evolving personalized interfaces the same way they design personalized feedback for each patient user. While designers currently are the ones to decide on the end-design of an AI solution, there is an expectation that the data generated from the users is going to be the determinant of what interfaces users see on their devices. This creates hurdles for the standarization and approval of evaluation metrics for machine-learning generated interfaces. These metrics not only need to satisfy conventional HCI criteria, but also need to account for new Human-AI interaction criteria (Kirsch 2017).

## 3.5 Foreseeing the Unforeseeable—Adapting to an Ever Changing Human-AI Interaction

As machine learning models are progressively learning to adapt to the unexpectancies of patients' behavior, the human-AI interaction is becoming more and more blurred (Adadi and Berrada 2018). This therefore requires expert designers to think further ahead to mitigate the risks of a swiftly developing AI. Medical systems that incorporate autonomous learning face the challenge of quickly adapting to the changes of medical notions and patients' feedback (Adadi and Berrada 2018). Therefore, the role of human-AI interaction in this case is of essential importance to serve as a mediator between the clinician and the AI to overcome those challenges. While the traditional HCI evaluation standards like visibility, feedback, constraints, mapping, affordances, and consistency (Norman 2002) are still relevant in the design of a system's interface, they remain not enough to examine machine learning systems that are user-adaptive.

# 4 Conclusion

To conclude, the past decade has witnessed an increase in processing power. This increase has lead to the availability of artificial intelligence for mainstream audiences. The accessibility of AI has provided a promise for incorporation in the medical field. However, attention has been drawn to the societal hurdles associated with these intelligent systems, especially with regards to how machine learning algorithms show failure of accuracy compared to the clinicians' expected standards, or how they disadvantage a certain category of patients over another depending on the data fed for training. Moreover, another hurdle challenging AI/ML systems is their black-box aspect. The opacity of the inner functioning of neural networks composing certain algorithms makes the task of understandablity, explainability, and improvement difficult to the clinicians. This leads them to being more unaware about the possibilities and capabilities of what a machine learning system can offer. From a Human-AI interaction standpoint, light has been shed on specifying a precise role that the human, being either a patient or a clinician, plays in the interaction equation. The challenge lies in how the user should be at the same time controlling the AI system, as well as working in tandem with it to improve the decision outcomes that are best for the patient.

# References

Adadi A, Berrada M (2018) Peeking inside the black-box: a survey on explainable artificial intelligence (XAI). IEEE Access 6:52138–52160. https://doi.org/10.1109/access.2018.2870052

Alber M, Tepole AB, Cannon WR, De S, Dura-Bernal S, Garikipati K, Karniadakis G, Lytton WW, Perdikaris P, Petzold L, Kuhl E (2019) Integrating machine learning and multiscale modeling–perspectives, challenges, and opportunities in the biological, biomedical, and behavioral sciences. Nat Partner J Digit Med 2(1):1–11. https://doi.org/10.1038/s41746-019-0193-y

Amershi S, Inkpen K, Teevan J, Kikin-Gil R, Horvitz E, Weld D, Vorvoreanu M, Fourney A, Nushi B, Collisson P, Suh J, Iqbal S, Bennett PN (2019)Guidelines for human-AI interaction. In: Proceedings of the 2019 CHI conference on human factors in computing systems—CHI 19. ACM Press. [Online]. Available: https://doi.org/10.1145/3290605.3300233

Amira A, Agoulmine N, Bensaali F, Bermak A, Dimitrakopoulos G (2019) Special issue: empowering eHealth with smart internet of things (IoT) medical devices. J Sens Act Netw 8(2):33. https://doi.org/10.3390/jsan8020033

Chancellor S, Lin Z, Goodman EL, Zerwas S, Choudhury MD (2016) Quantifying and predicting mental illness severity in online pro-eating disorder communities. In: Proceedings of the 19th ACM conference on computer-supported cooperative work & social computing—CSCW 16. ACM Press. [Online]. Available: https://doi.org/10.1145/2818048.2819973

Dove G, Halskov K, Forlizzi J, Zimmerman J (2017) UX design innovation. In: Proceedings of the 2017 CHI conference on human factors in computing systems - CHI 17. ACM Press. [Online]. Available: https://doi.org/10.1145/3025453.3025739

Dwork C, Hardt M, Pitassi T, Reingold O, Zemel R (2012) Fairness through awareness. In: Proceedings of the 3rd innovations in theoretical computer science conference on—ITCS 12. ACM Press. [Online]. Available: https://doi.org/10.1145/2090236.2090255

Fernandez-Luque L, Aupetit M, Palotti J, Singh M, Fadlelbari A, Baggag A, Khowaja K, Al-Thani D (2019) Health lifestyle data-driven applications using pervasive computing. In: Big data, big challenges: a healthcare perspective. Springer International Publishing, pp 115–126. [Online]. Available: https://doi.org/10.1007/978-3-030-06109-8_10

Fogg BJ (2002) Persuasive technology: using computers to change what we think and do. Ubiquity 2002:2. [Online]. Available: https://doi.org/10.1145/764008.763957

Gillies M, Lee B, dAlessandro N, Tilmanne J, Kulesza T, Caramiaux B, Fiebrink R, Tanaka A, Garcia J, Bevilacqua F, Heloir A, Nunnari F, Mackay W, Amershi S (2016) Human-centred machine learning. In: Proceedings of the 2016 CHI conference extended abstracts on human factors in computing systems - CHI EA 16. ACM Press. [Online]. Available: https://doi.org/10.1145/2851581.2856492

In: Proceedings of the conference on fairness, accountability, and transparency, FAT* 2019, Atlanta, GA, USA, 29–31 Jan 2019. ACM. [Online]. Available: https://dl.acm.org/citation.cfm?id=3287588

Inkpen K, Chancellor S, Choudhury MD, Veale M, Baumer EPS (2019) Where is the human? In: Extended abstracts of the 2019 conference on human factors in computing systems CHI—EA 19. ACM Press. [Online]. Available: https://doi.org/10.1145/3290607.3299002

Khowaja K, Banire B, Al-Thani D, Sqalli MT, Aqle A, Shah A, Salim SS (2020) Augmented reality for learning of children and adolescents with autism spectrum disorder (asd): A systematic review. IEEE Access 8:78779–78807

Kirsch A (2017) Explain to whom? Putting the user in the center of explainable AI. In: Proceedings of the first international workshop on comprehensibility and explanation in AI and ML 2017 co-located with 16th international conference of the italian association for artificial intelligence (AI*IA 2017), Bari, Italy. [Online]. Available: https://hal.archives-ouvertes.fr/hal-01845135

Koh H, Tan G (2005) Data mining applications in healthcare. J Healthc Inf Manage JHIM 19:64–72

Kurabe K, Kato Y, Koike M, Jinno K, Yamashita K, Kito K, Sqalli MT, Tatsuno K (2016) A robot controller for power distribution line maintenance robot working by task-level command,, In:

2016 IEEE/SICE international symposium on system integration (SII). IEEE. [Online]. Available: https://doi.org/10.1109/sii.2016.7844038

Lazer D, Kennedy R, King G, Vespignani A (2014) The parable of google flu: traps in big data analysis. Science 343(6176):1203–1205. https://doi.org/10.1126/science.1248506

Marvel FA, Wang J, Martin SS (2018) Digital health innovation: a toolkit to navigate from concept to clinical testing. JMIR Cardio 2(1):e2. [Online]. Available: https://doi.org/10.2196/cardio.7586

Norman DA (2002) The design of everyday things. Basic Books Inc, New York, NY, USA

Olteanu A, Castillo C, Diaz F, Kıcıman E (2019) Social data: biases, methodological pitfalls, and ethical boundaries. Front Big Data 2. [Online]. Available: https://doi.org/10.3389/fdata.2019.00013

Pedreschi D, Giannotti F, Guidotti R, Monreale A, Ruggieri S, Turini F (2019) eaningful explanations of black box AI decision systems. In: Proceedings of the AAAI conference on artificial intelligence, vol 33, pp 9780–9784. [Online]. Available: https://doi.org/10.1609/aaai.v33i01.33019780

Piwek L, Ellis DA, Andrews S, Joinson A (2016) The rise of consumer health wearables: promises and barriers. PLOS Med 13(2):e1001953. https://doi.org/10.1371/journal.pmed.1001953

Shah P, Kendall F, Khozin S, Goosen R, Hu J, Laramie J, Ringel M, Schork N (2019) Artificial intelligence and machine learning in clinical development: a translational perspective. Nat Partner J Digit Med 2(1). https://doi.org/10.1038/s41746-019-0148-3

Sqalli MT, Al-Thani D (2019) AI-supported health coaching model for patients with chronic diseases. In: 2019 16th International symposium on wireless communication systems (ISWCS). IEEE [Online]. Available: https://doi.org/10.1109/ISWCS.2019.8877113

Sqalli MT, Tatsuno K, Kurabe K, Ando H, Obitsu H, Itakura R, Aoto T, Yoshino K (2016) Improvement of a tele-presence robot autonomous navigation using SLAM algorithm. In: 2016 International symposium on micro-nanomechatronics and human science (MHS). IEEE. [Online]. Available: https://doi.org/10.1109/mhs.2016.7824221

Turakhia MP, Desai M, Hedlin H, Rajmane A, Talati N, Ferris T, Desai S, Nag D, Patel M, Kowey P, Rumsfeld JS, Russo AM, Hills MT, Granger CB, Mahaffey KW, Perez MV (2019) Rationale and design of a large-scale, app-based study to identify cardiac arrhythmias using a smartwatch: the apple heart study. Am Heart J 207:66–75. https://doi.org/10.1016/j.ahj.2018.09.002

Wiegand T, Krishnamurthy R, Kuglitsch M, Lee N, Pujari S, Salathé M, Wenzel M, Xu S (2019) WHO and ITU establish benchmarking process for artificial intelligence in health. The Lancet 394(10192):9–11. https://doi.org/10.1016/s0140-6736(19)30762-7

Wilbanks JT, Topol EJ (2016) Stop the privatization of health data. Nat Int Weekly J Sci 535

Yamashita K, Kato Y, Kurabe K, Koike M, Jinno K, Kito K, Tatsuno K, Sqalli MT (2016) Remote operation of a robot for maintaining electric power distribution system using a joystick and a master arm as a human robot interface medium. In: 2016 International symposium on micro-nanomechatronics and human science (MHS). IEEE. [Online]. Available: https://doi.org/10.1109/mhs.2016.7824229

Yang Q, Scuito A, Zimmerman J, Forlizzi J, Steinfeld A (2018) Investigating how experienced UX designers effectively work with machine learning. In: Proceedings of the 2018 on designing interactive systems conference 2018 - DIS 18. ACM Press. [Online]. Available: https://doi.org/10.1145/3196709.3196730

# Artificial Intelligence in Healthcare from a Policy Perspective

**Monica Aggarwal, Christian Gingras, and Raisa Deber**

**Abstract** The growth of Artificial Intelligence (AI) technologies in health care is driving a growing recognition among policymakers, businesses and researchers that there is a need for policies to address certain potential consequences of AI innovation. In this chapter, we provide insight on several policy implications and challenges relating to the impact of AI on accuracy, fairness and transparency, data privacy and consent, accountability, and workforce disruption. These issues include: monitoring of accuracy; minimizing bias and encouraging transparency, ensuring appropriate use, assessment of who is receiving the information and how it is being used, protecting privacy through data protection requirements, enactment of laws that defines accountabilities, establishment of policies for labour disruption; implementation of professional standards and codes of conduct; adapting educational training for clinicians; and determining what technologies will be insured and funded. Additional complexities arise when AI crosses geographic boundaries. The design, development and implementation of policy and regulation should be in conjunction with a diversity of stakeholders including product developers, researchers, patients, health care providers and policymakers.

**Keywords** Artificial intelligence · Policy · Regulation · Ethics · Algorithm bias · Privacy · Consent · Accountability · Human resources

## 1 Introduction

Artificial Intelligence (AI) is a branch of computer science concerned with the development of systems that can perform tasks that usually require human intelligence,

M. Aggarwal (✉)
Dalla Lana School of Public Health, University of Toronto, Toronto, Canada
e-mail: monica.aggarwal@utoronto.ca

C. Gingras
Innovative Health Care Management Solutions Inc., Toronto, Canada

R. Deber
Institute of Health Policy, Management and Evaluation, University of Toronto, Toronto, Canada

© Springer Nature Switzerland AG 2021
M. Househ et al. (eds.), *Multiple Perspectives on Artificial Intelligence in Healthcare*,
Lecture Notes in Bioengineering, https://doi.org/10.1007/978-3-030-67303-1_5

such as problem-solving, reasoning, and recognition (An Overview of Clinical Applications of Artificial Intelligence 2018). AI has significant prospect to fundamentally transform the delivery of health care. Despite the significant potential of AI, there are several policy challenges that need to be considered by policymakers as they embark on the AI journey.

Analyzing the policy implications is complex, because AI is not homogeneous (Scherer 2016), and the policy issues may vary accordingly. AI has been suggested for a wide variety of tasks, including but not restricted to assisting in health data management (including streamlining administrative processes to facilitate quality assurance); searching the medical literature in specialized domains; assisting in repetitive jobs (such as analyzing radiology images); smart algorithms to help interpret tests, improve diagnostics and generate targeted treatment pathway design; and patient empowerment (including allowing self-monitoring patient management) (Mesko 2017). The policy implications accordingly may vary depending on what the goals of the AI are, and who it is serving.

Policy can be defined as "a set of interrelated decisions taken by a political actor or group of actors concerning the selection of goals and the means of achieving them within a specified situation where these decisions should, in principle, be within the power of these actors to achieve" (Jenkins 1978). Policy makers can use a variety of policy instruments to accomplish this, which may include exhortation (providing information), expenditure (subsidizing activities), regulation, or public ownership (Doern and Phidd 1992). As these definitions recognize, there is likely to be significant variation in who would be responsible for these policy decisions, and the policy instruments they could use.

The growth of AI technologies in health care is driving the growing recognition among policymakers, businesses and researchers that there is a need for the establishment of policies to address the consequences of AI innovation. Several countries have released strategies to encourage the use and development of AI (Dutton 2018; OECD 2019). A number of approaches are being used to regulate AI, including: encouraging AI actors to develop self-regulatory mechanisms such as codes of conduct, accountability standards, ethical frameworks and best practices; and establishing public- and private-sector oversight mechanisms in the form of compliance reviews, audits, conformity assessments and certification schemes for AI applications (OECD 2019).

The purpose of this chapter is to provide insight to policymakers, researchers, businesses, clinicians, patients and caregivers on the policy implications and challenges relating to the impact of AI on such issues as: accuracy, fairness and transparency, data privacy and consent, accountability, and workforce disruption. Table 1 provides an overview of some challenges and opportunities.

**Table 1** Challenges and opportunities

| Challenges | Opportunities |
|---|---|
| Lack of universal definition of AI | Jurisdiction establish a consensus-based definition of AI amongst all stakeholders for the purpose of designing AI Policy and Regulation |
| Risk related to AI is unknown and algorithms are continually adapting and changing. | Basic "rules" anchored in Ethics are developed to allow for adaptability as AI risks and capabilities evolve |
| AI can discriminate due to algorithm bias or training data bias | Several approaches can be used to minimize the risk of discrimination. This includes: awareness building; funding development of representative datasets, organizational diversity policies and practices; recruitment of developers from diverse background; local and international standards (including post-market monitoring); technical solutions to detect and correct algorithmic bias; self-regulatory or regulatory approaches, and ethical governance and standards, and ethical auditing |
| Deep learning and Machine learning result in lack of transparency | Establish regulation and policies that articulates how transparency will be handled for consumers/patients. |
| Legal framework does not exist for who is accountable when harm is caused by autonomous AI applications | Laws must be developed in which there are multiple options for consideration:<br>1 – Establish AI as a "Person" under the law<br>2 – Introduce Enterprise Liability, assigning responsibility to all group involved in the creating and implementation of AI<br>3 – Modify duties of care of Health Professional to take into account AI and for them to exercise due care in its application |
| Privacy legislation is not well established around the globe. In the absence of laws and policies, significant investment may be invalidated once a framework is updated | Establish appropriate Policy and Regulation of AI to establish rules of engagement for the development of AI |
| AI challenges the traditional concept of consent | Establish guidelines for health care providers and private Companies on rules around the use of data and providing patients (or consumers) with information on the potential uses of their data |
| Fear of work displacement | Establish clear policies in the event that employment is displaced by AI function (i.e.: retraining programs, employment insurance, alternative taxation, etc...) |
| Adoption of AI in health care depend upon acceptance by health care professionals | Engage health care professional in discussions involving policy, product development and provide clinicians with education on the benefits and limitations of AI and how to use it. |

# 2 Artificial Intelligence Policy

Ideally, AI policy would maximize AI innovation and benefits, and minimize its potential costs and risk. Achieving the appropriate balance is not obvious, and may depend on the priorities of different decision makers.

AI software is viewed by regulatory bodies such as Health Canada and the FDA as a medical device (Jaremko et al. 2019). Accordingly, an intended use statement must be submitted by the device manufacturer to receive approval (Jaremko et al. 2019). If approved, the regulatory body can place additional controls on the device to ensure safety. In this case, liability rests with the health care practitioner using that device (Jaremko et al. 2019). An important delineator in legal and regulatory risk assessments is whether AI acts independently (i.e., the software makes diagnostic or treatment decisions that are automatically implemented or that the human user is not able to evaluate) or whether it augments or supports clinical decision-making (i.e., the software makes recommendations but the final decisions are made by a clinician) (Sullivan and Schweikart 2019). However, current legal standards and doctrines regarding medical malpractice are not always clear on where responsibilities should lie when AI supports or autonomously delivers healthcare services (Sullivan and Schweikart 2019).

One question is who the intended user of the AI will be. Much of AI could be viewed as an extension of existing technology. If a physician orders diagnostic testing (including imaging or laboratory tests), they would normally be returned with an interpretation of what these results mean. For such applications, similar regulatory controls would presumably exist, including ensuring that the test is being performed accurately, that the results are valid, and that the receiving provider understands the limitations of the test results and is responsible for communicating with the patients and ensuring that they understand the meaning of the results, and of the treatments that may be suggested. Such uses of AI do not represent significant new policy challenges.

To the extent that AI goes beyond such current testing, however, new issues may arise. One set of issues may result if the test results are provided to users other than clinicians. This may resemble such current examples as genetic tests provided to patients who order them on-line; there is a considerable literature about the potential risks to patients of receiving inaccurate information. Similarly, test results may be provided to employers (who may use them to discharge employees), insurers (who may use them to deny coverage or increase premiums), etc.

Another set of issues arises if the AI provider is not in the same jurisdiction as the recipient. While this can be advantageous (e.g., to patients in rural/remote areas without the infrastructure to provide such tests), it can also be problematic to the extent that it is unclear who will set and enforce the regulations to ensure that the tests are accurate, and that other ethical and regulatory issues are complied with.

Currently, there are two main approaches used for the regulation of AI that represent different balances between encouraging innovation, and avoiding risks. The European Union (EU) has adopted the "precautionary principle" (Thierer et al. 2017) approach which imposes limits or bans on certain applications due to their potential risks (Pesapane et al. 2018). The European regulatory regime is based on three directives on medical devices in which it requires manufacturers to ensure that the devices they produce are fit for their intended purpose and they comply with the requirements set out by the directives (Pesapane et al. 2018). This assessment can take place by the manufacturer or by a notified body, which is an independent accredited certification organization appointed by the EU Member States (Pesapane et al. 2018). On the other hand, the United States has adopted the "permissionless" innovation approach (Thierer et al. 2017; Pesapane et al. 2018) which permits experimentation with the expectation that issues will be addressed as they arise. The Food and Drug Administration (FDA) categorizes the medical devices into three classes, according to their uses and risks, in which the degree of regulation increases with more risk (Allen 2019). These approaches are hotly debated since the "precautionary principle" approach is seen to inhibit innovation and the "permissionless" approach is seen to increase risk of harm. The consensus appears to be that an ideal approach would be one that is a balance between these approaches.

Examples of policy issues in AI include: accuracy, fairness and transparency; data privacy and consent; accountability, and workforce disruption.

# 3   Accuracy, Fairness and Transparency

A substantial body of AI literature draws attention to the potential for bias by AI applications towards certain population sub-groups, which can result in discrimination, inequality and marginalization. In machine learning, algorithms rely on multiple data sets, or training data, that are used to make predictions about the 'correct' answer for the patient/client (An Overview of Clinical Applications of Artificial Intelligence 2018; Bathaee 2018). To the extent that this data is biased, incomplete or inaccurate, the AI can produce similarly biased results (An Overview of Clinical Applications of Artificial Intelligence 2018; Bathaee 2018). This can lead to decisions which can have a collective, disparate impact on certain groups of people even without the programmer's intention to discriminate (Lee et al. 2019).

One example is a recent study in a US hospital, that showed how the use of algorithms to identify primary care patients with the most complex needs (who would then be selected for the hospital's complex care program) discriminated against black patients (Obermeyer et al. 2019). The software attempted to predict patients' future health needs, but used their future health costs as a proxy for their health needs. Because Blacks generated lower cost due to structural inequalities in the health care system, they were less likely to be selected (Obermeyer et al. 2019). This example raises important policy questions about how we ensure data is representative so machine learning algorithms are generalizable, what mechanisms should be used to minimize discriminatory bias (e.g., antidiscrimination laws, consumer protection, industry standards), and what incentives should be in place to develop and adopt best practices? (Calo 2017).

The literature suggests several approaches to prevent algorithm discrimination. Industry standards can shape self-regulation, co-regulation and setting of regulatory requirements (OECD 2019; Lee et al. 2019). Ethical governance and standards can be used to clearly define the principles of 'fairness (OECD 2019). Building awareness of discriminatory practices (OECD 2019) and recruiting developers from diverse backgrounds permits representation of a range of populations (OECD 2019; Lee et al. 2019). Finally, simulation of predictions and using technical solutions to detect and correct algorithmic bias can be used before implementation (OECD 2019).

Many of these depend heavily upon the desire of the AI producers to ensure accuracy, rather than on the actions of regulators.

Another important policy issue arises from the lack of transparency with respect to the decisions made by deep learning technology. From a policy perspective, transparency focuses on how a decision is made, who participates in the process and the factors used to make the decision (OECD 2019). For example, some 'black box' machine learning models used in medical diagnosis are quite accurate at predicting the probability of a medical condition, but have been described as being too complex for humans to understand, which also means that errors are harder to detect (OECD 2019). There has been significant movement to make AI applications more explainable, but this can sacrifice accuracy if this requires reducing the variables to a set small enough for humans to understand (OECD 2019). In such cases, the potential harms and benefits from these different types of models need to be weighed to see how we ensure that black-box algorithms are high quality and safe, and how much confidence we will place in treatment recommendations based on complex or 'black box' algorithms, particularly when new variables arise that may not be incorporated in that model.

In Europe, the General Data Protection Regulation (GDPR) provides individuals with the "right not to be subject to a decision based solely on automated means" (Nuffield Council on Bioethics 2018). The regulation also specifies that individuals should also be provided with meaningful information about how automated systems make their decisions (Nuffield Council on Bioethics 2018; Mowat Centre 2019). However, the scope and content of these restrictions—for example, whether and how AI can be intelligible—and how they will apply in the United Kingdom, remain uncertain and contested (Nuffield Council on Bioethics 2018). In Canada, the federal government has developed a set of guiding principles for the responsible use of AI and a Directive on Automated Decision-Making (Mowat Centre 2019).

## 4   Data Privacy and Consent

Because AI technologies involve the use of large datasets, there are also policy issues related to data privacy and consumer consent (Deane 2018). The expectations with respect to privacy varies around the world, particularly when these are anchored in cultural beliefs and moral judgments (Adler 1991). There are also differences in whether one is dealing with de-identified data that is used to construct the algorithms, or the personal data associated with an individual patient. A comparison of four commonly recognized healthcare privacy standards (Organisation for Economic Co-operation and Development Privacy Principles, Generally Accepted Privacy Principles, Personal Information Protection and Electronic Documents Act, Data Protection Act) indicates that all of these standards encompass principles that are premised on consent, collection, disclosure, access, security, quality, accountability, transparency, proportionality, notice and notification (Virtue and Rainey 2015).

A related set of policy issues relate to who is collecting (and using) the data. In some cases, regulations, policies and frameworks explicitly specify which entities are "covered" or "not covered" by these privacy rules. For example, under the US Health Insurance Portability and Accountability Act (HIPAA), physicians, health insurers, medical providers are "covered entities" while large companies such as Google, Apple are not. This means that a physician collecting a patient's data on heart rate will be subject to HIPAA but the same information collected by a private company such as Apple (e.g., via the Apple Watch), will not be (Price and Nicholson 2017). The EU is the only jurisdiction that has regulation via data protection legislation via the GDPR, which is applicable to all data regardless of who owns it (Forcier et al. 2019). The EU has also published new guidelines on developing ethical AI which include seven basic requirements; these include Privacy and Data Governance, which specifically guarantees privacy and data protection during the entire AI lifecycle (Commission and Ethics Guidelines for Trustworthy AI 2019). In some instance, these regulations have been successful in addressing breaches in consent. For example, an AI program, Google DeepMind, was provided with patient records from Royal Free Hospital in the United Kingdom without patient consent. The information had sensitive information about HIV status, mental health history and abortion. The Royal Free argued during the trial that they had "implied consent" because the patients were aware that the app offered "direct care". The Information Commissioners Office (ICO) ruled that the deal was illegal but did not fine the hospital or Google (Duhigg 2012).

A related ethical issue with respect to privacy results if a predictive analytics model is used to create personal health information using information from individuals such as their location, purchase patterns, and/or internet access, without their consent or awareness (Deane 2018). In 2012, it was revealed that the Target stores in the US used big data and an AI algorithm to predict whether a customer was pregnant; the algorithm estimated due date based on the purchase habits associated with 25 products, and was used to send coupons for diapers and other pregnancy/parenting related coupons to these targeted consumers. When it was discovered that the enterprise was engaged in this activity, Target did not stop the practice but instead introduced additional random coupon offerings to the customer.(Reuters 2018) This was legal under HIPAA rules, because Target was not a "covered entity" as defined by the Act, but did present ethical issues related to consent, particularly if the consumers had not formally agreed to share their information with Target, and/or did not realize this information could be used to accurately predict a medical condition. This example also touches on personal data ownership and who owns it and how is it protected. For example, what would be th consequence if an employer discovered this information and discriminated against the individual by terminating their job, or if insurers changed coverage?

A related ethical issue that is relevant to the principles of consent, collection and disclosure and access is related to who is provided with the data? For example, there are examples of insurance companies that are moving towards interactive policy with "optional" fitness tracking in which refusing to participate in the voluntary program results in higher prices (framed in terms of not receiving discounts) (Caruana, et al. 2015). This example raises similar questions about what constitutes consumer consent, as well as what happens to the data. If AI data indicates that consumers are at high risk, their rates may rise, or they may become uninsurable. Can the data be deleted on the request of the consumer? Can the company use the information to predict clusters of high-risk consumers and adjust their rates? Should there be compensation to the consumers if their data is used by the insurer for economic gain? How do we prevent insurers from cherry-picking clients?

Many of these issues are not currently addressed in many privacy acts around the world. Given the cultural expectations with respect to privacy are locally driven, some policy analysts suggest that jurisdictions should develop their own local policy and regulatory framework, while others may propose more general frameworks. Issues that these frameworks would need to consider include which organizations would be included (e.g., health care providers? Insurers? Employers? Any organizations with health care data?), what mechanisms will be in place to ensure that product vendors are creating AI applications that are aligned with privacy and consent rules and are complying with the policy and regulatory frameworks, and how consumers will be educated and informed by all data collecting organizations about how their data is being used.

# 5 Accountability

In most jurisdictions, there are regulatory structures in place to ensure that clinicians try to make accurate decisions. To the extent that clinicians receive the data from AI, they have some responsibility for evaluating its recommendations. However, the lack of transparency in 'black box' decision-making and its potential to cause medical errors may raise legal questions about what happens when a black-box AI system makes an erroneous diagnosis that results in harm to the patient? One study found that the use of machine learning to predict the risk of hospital attendants to develop pneumonia resulted in instructing physicians to send high-risk pneumonia patients home (Ardila et al. 2019). In this case, what happens if a patient dies because treatment was not provided? Who is legally responsible for this error? When should the responsibility be with the health care practitioner, health care organization, product vendor or the machine itself? Should this be a joint accountability? On the other hand, what are the implications for medical malpractice when a health care provider rejects diagnosis or recommendations from a machine?

The determination of liability regarding the use of the system and the user need further definition and clarification (Sullivan and Schweikart 2019; Reddy et al. 2019). Experts have offered possible solutions for current law or legal doctrines. One option for consideration is to implement AI personhood, which views the machine as an independent "person" under the law with duties who can then be sued directly for negligence claims (Sullivan and Schweikart 2019). In such instances, the AI system will be required to be insured and such claims will be paid out from the insurance. The second is to introduce common enterprise liability, which assigns responsibility to all groups involved in the use and implementation of the AI system (Sullivan and Schweikart 2019). The third solution is to modify the duties and standard of care of health care professionals using black-box AI that would require facilities and health care professionals to exercise due care in evaluating and implementing black-box algorithms (Sullivan and Schweikart 2019). Under this model, health care professionals are responsible for harm if they did not take adequate measures in properly evaluating the black-box AI technologies used in caring for the patient. Additional complications may arise if the AI is in a different jurisdiction, and hence not bound by the regulatory or legal requirements in place where the damage occurred.

# 6    Workforce Disruption

AI has the potential not only to be more accurate, but to work faster than humans. Several new studies have shown that computers can outperform physicians in cancer screenings and disease diagnoses (Rodriguez-Ruiz et al. 2019; Sharkey and Sharkey 2012). Others argue that AI can help streamline administrative processes, provide bots to help patients manage alone (e.g., reminding them to take their medicine), and better match patients with optimal treatment (Mesko 2017). There is a literature expressing concerns about whether AI will displace jobs for health care professionals by mastering tasks currently performed by people, and/or result in the employment of less skilled staff (SVayena et al. 2018). To the extent that AI is used to replace human contact, this may raise concerns (Secretary of State for Health and Social Care 2019). Others argue that this will free professionals from repetitive tasks and enable them to spend more of their time with patients (OECD 2019). Furthermore, AI is unlikely to have the capacity to understand emotions and show compassion, components that are foundational to the patient-health care professional relationship and heavily valued by patients and their families (Reddy et al. 2019). Given the potential impact to the workforce, it'll be important for governments to implement policies for managing this transition.

However, the fear of losing jobs can have implications for the adoption of AI by health care professionals. If there is a perception that health care professionals will be replaced, it is less likely that they will wish to adopt AI innovation. This raises ethical issues of whether medical establishments should be allowed to block AI technologies that are proven to be safer, better, or cheaper but may threaten jobs? Even if health care professionals adopt the 'black box' technology there is also the risk that reliance on a machine's decisions will reduce their skills or make them complacent, and might impact the patient-health care professional relationship if the clinician cannot explain the decision to the patient. This also raises concerns on the impact this will have on patient decision-making processes.

Another set of issues relate to who pays for these AI applications. To the extent that these applications are developed by for-profit industries seeking to maximize profits, there is a market for services provided directly to patients (and/or employers and insurers), many of which will not be covered by insurance. This category of applications is also less likely to undergo scrutiny by clinicians to assess their accuracy. At present, they may not be subject to regulatory processes. There is also the issue of who will pay for AI technology in health care organizations and physician offices, whether insurers would only pay for AI driven recommendations, and, if AI technology reduces the time spent by physicians to make treatment decisions, whether it should impact their compensation model.

As the industry develops AI applications, it will be important to maintain trust, which may require involving clinicians and patients in their design and development. Revision of professional standards and codes of conduct to accommodate changes from AI may also be required, as well as modification of education and training systems to skill and re-skill health care professionals to work in this new environment

(Dutton 2018). Policymakers will need to determine what AI technologies will be insured and funded. In addition, patient literacy with respect to the limitations of AI will also be important (Reddy et al. 2019).

## 7 Conclusions

The need for regulation of AI will continue to grow as more and more AI technologies are released in health care. Regulatory policy will need to balance the risk of stifling innovation by overregulation with the risk of harm caused by under-regulation. AI policy will need to focus on regulation that: monitors the accuracy of the recommendations proposed by the AI application, ensures that it is being used appropriately, minimizes bias and encourages transparency, assesses who is receiving the information and how it is being used, protects privacy through data protection requirements, enacts laws that clearly define accountabilities, establishes policies for labour disruption; implements professional standards and codes of conduct; adapts educational training to skill health care professionals; and determines what AI technologies will be insured and funded for clinicians. To the extent that these AI applications cross geographic boundaries, there are also questions about who will regulate them, and how. Development of regulation needs to be informed in conjunction with a diversity of stakeholders including product developers, researchers, patients, health care providers and policymakers.

As jurisdictions develop regulatory frameworks, it will be imperative that all stakeholders across sectors are engaged in the development and review of regulation and compliance requirements for new digital healthcare technologies.

## References

Adler MJ (1991) Desires right & wrong: the ethics of enough. Macmillan Publishing Company

Allen B (2019) The Role of the FDA in ensuring the safety and efficacy of artificial intelligence software and devices. J Am Coll Radiol 16(2):208–210

An Overview of Clinical Applications of Artificial Intelligence (2018) CADTH, Ottawa (CADTH issues in emerging health technologies; issue 174). Retrieved from: https://www.cadth.ca/sites/default/files/pdf/eh0070_overview_clinical_applications_of_AI.pdf

Ardila D, Kiraly AP, Bharadwaj S, Choi B, Reicher JJ (2019) End-to-end lung cancer screening with three-dimensional deep learning on low-dose chest computed tomography. Nat Med 25:954–961

Bathaee Y (2018) The artificial intelligence black box and the failure of intent and causation. Harvard J Law Technol 31(2). https://jolt.law.harvard.edu/assets/articlePDFs/v31/The-Artificial-Intelligence-Black-Box-and-the-Failure-of-Intent-and-Causation-Yavar-Bathaee.pdf. Accessed 13 Sep 2019

Calo R (2017) Artificial intelligence policy: a primer and roadmap. https://lawreview.law.ucdavis.edu/issues/51/2/Symposium/51-2_Calo.pdf. Accessed 01 Sept 2019

Caruana R et al (2015) Intelligible models for healthcare. In: Proceedings of the 21th ACM SIGKDD international conference on knowledge discovery and data mining, pp 1721–30. http://people. dbmi.columbia.edu/noemie/papers/15kdd.pdf

Deane M (2018) AI and the future of privacy. https://towardsdatascience.com/ai-and-the-future-of-privacy-3d5f6552a7c4. Accessed 15 Oct 2019

Doern GB, Phidd RW (1992) Canadian public policy: Ideas, structure, process, 2nd edn. Nelson, Toronto, ON

Duhigg C (2012) How company learn your secrets. The New York Times Magazine. https://www.nytimes.com/2012/02/19/magazine/shopping-habits.html. Accessed 12 Oct 2019

Dutton T (2018) An overview of national AI strategies. Retrieved from https://medium.com/politics-ai/an-overview-of-national-ai-strategies-2a70ec6edfdOECD (2019), Artificial Intelligence in Society, OECD Publishing, Paris. https://doi.org/10.1787/eedfee77-en

European Commission (2019) Ethics guidelines for trustworthy AI. (https://ec.europa.eu/digital-single-market/en/news/ethics-guidelines-trustworthy-ai). Accessed 12 Oct 2019

Forcier MB, Gallois H, Mullan S, Joly Y (2019) Integrating artificial intelligence into health care through data access: can the GDPR act as a beacon for policymakers? J Law Biosci, pp 317–335. https://doi.org/10.1093/jlb/lsz013

Jaremko JL, Azar M, Bromwich R, Lum A, Alicia Cheong LH, Gilbert M et al (2019) Canadian association of radiologists white paper on ethical and legal issues related to artificial intelligence in radiology. Can Assoc Radiol J 70(2):107–118. https://doi.org/10.1016/j.carj.2019.03.001. Epub 5 Apr 2019

Jenkins WI (1978) Policy analysis: a political and organizational perspective. Martin's Press, New York, St

Lee NT, Resnick P, Barton G (2019) Algorithmic bias detection mitigation: Best practices and policies to reduce consumer harm. https://www.brookings.edu/research/algorithmic-bias-detection-and-mitigation-best-practices-and-policies-to-reduce-consumer-harms/. Accessed 20 Sept 2019

Mesko B (2017) A guide to artificial intelligence in healthcare

Mowat Centre (2019) Governing the future: creating standards for artificial intelligence and algorithms. https://munkschool.utoronto.ca/mowatcentre/governing-the-future-creating-standards-for-artificial-intelligence-and-algorithms/. Accessed 12 Oct 2019

Nuffield Council on Bioethics (2018) Artificial intelligence in healthcare and research. https://nuffieldbioethics.org/wp-content/uploads/Artificial-Intelligence-AI-in-healthcare-and-research.pdf. Accessed 30 Oct 2019

Obermeyer Z, Powers B, Vogeli C, Mullainathan S (2019) Dissecting racial bias in an algorithm used to manage the health of populations. Science 366(6464):447–453. https://doi.org/10.1126/science.aax2342

OECD (2019) Artificial intelligence in society. OECD Publishing, Paris. https://doi.org/10.1787/eedfee77-en

Pesapane F, Volonté C, Codari, M, Sardanelli F(2018). Artificial intelligence as a medical device in radiology: ethical and regulatory issues in Europe and the United States. Insights Imag 9(5):745–753

Price W, Nicholson II (2017) Artificial intelligence in health care: applications and legal implications. SciTech Lawyer 14 (1). https://repository.law.umich.edu/cgi/viewcontent.cgi?article=2932&context=articles

Reddy S, Allan, S, Coghlan S, Cooper P (2019) A governance model for the application of AI in health Care. J Am Med Inf Assoc, pp 1–7. https://doi.org/10.1093/jamia/ocz192

Reuters T (2018) All John Hancock life insurance policies to include fitness incentives. CBC. https://www.vmmed.com/blog/all-john-hancock-life-insurance-policies-to-include-fitness-incentives/. Accessed 12 Oct 2019

Rodriguez-Ruiz A, Lång K, Gubern-Merida A, Broeders M, Gennaro G et al (2019) Stand-alone artificial intelligence for breast cancer detection in mammography: comparison with 101 radiologists. JNCI J Natl Cancer Inst 111(9):916–922

Scherer MU (2016). Regulating artificial intelligence systems: risks, challenges, competencies and strategies. Harvard J Law Technol 29(2). http://jolt.law.harvard.edu/articles/pdf/v29/29HarvJLT ech353.pdf. Accessed 12 Nov 2019

Secretary of State for Health and Social Care (2019) Topol review: preparing the healthcare workforce to deliver the digital future. https://pharmafield.co.uk/healthcare/the-topol-review-prepar ing-the-healthcare-workforce-to-deliver-the-digital-future/. Accessed 15 Oct 2019

Sharkey A, Sharkey N (2012) Granny and the robots: ethical issues in robot care for the elderly. Ethics Inf Technol 14:27–40

Sullivan HR, Schweikart SJ (2019) Are current tort liability doctrines adequate for addressing injury caused by AI. AMA J Ethics 21(2): E160–166. https://doi.org/10.1001/amajethics.2019.160

SVayena E, Blasimme A, Cohen IG (2018) Machine learning in medicine: addressing ethical challenges. PLoS Med 15(11): e1002689. https://doi.org/10.1371/journal.pmed.1002689

Telegraph (2016, 4 May) Royal free breached UK data law in 1.6m patient deal with Googl's DeepMind. https://www.theguardian.com/technology/2016/may/04/google-deepmind-access-healthcare-data-patients

Thierer A, O'Sullivan A, Russel R (2017) Artificial intelligence and public policy. Mercatus Research Paper. Available via https://www.mercatus.org/system/files/thierer-artificial-intellige nce-policy-mr-mercatus-v1.pdf

Virtue T, Rainey J (2015) HCISPP study guide. Syngress Publishing

# Privacy-Preserving AI in Healthcare

**Saif Al-Kuwari**

**Abstract** Recent advances in Artificial Intelligence promise a brighter future for many industries. Particularly, in healthcare, AI is now playing a central role to complement understanding of the current problems while paving the way for new discoveries. However, as AI is fueled by data, serious concerns are rising to keep the balance between expanding AI and preserving the privacy of the data it utilizes, which, in the case of healthcare, often contains personal and sensitive information. In this chapter, we shed some light on how to preserve the privacy of data in healthcare while still harnessing and optimizing AI. We discuss several technical solutions that enable AI to advance while preserving the privacy of the underlying data. We also discuss privacy from a legal point of view and show how traditional legislation may fail to provide adequate protection to health data, then discuss more recent legislations with promising approach to achieving adequate data privacy.

**Keywords** Health data · Privacy-preserving · Healthcare · AI · Privacy

## 1 Introduction

Artificial Intelligence (AI) continues to change many aspects of our lives. Generally, AI attempts to perform tasks that typically require human intelligence, such as decision, prediction and classification based tasks. While its applications have only recently hyped, AI is not a new concept. In fact, the ideas and applications of AI have been studies and discussed as early as the 1960s by pioneers such as Oliver Selfridge and Claude Shannon. However, back then, AI has unfortunately failed to sustain. The early days of AI were not as bright as most were hoping for. Results were not very promising, and algorithms were extremely inefficient. After a reasonably long wait, funders have already given up on AI, and decided to cut all investments. That was the beginning of what is known as *The AI Winter*. Around 2010, interest in AI has suddenly refueled. It turns out the problem of the 1960s AI was not the technology

S. Al-Kuwari (✉)
College of Science and Engineering, Hamad Bin Khalifa University, Doha, Qatar
e-mail: smalkuwari@hbku.edu.qa

© Springer Nature Switzerland AG 2021
M. Househ et al. (eds.), *Multiple Perspectives on Artificial Intelligence in Healthcare*,
Lecture Notes in Bioengineering, https://doi.org/10.1007/978-3-030-67303-1_6

itself, but rather the resources that were required to unlock its potential, namely: data and computational power. While computational power has certainly played a major role in reviving AI, it was data which enabled AI to make all the breakthroughs we see today.

Unfortunately, the fact that AI is being driven by data raises concerns about privacy of that data. The situation is exacerbated when such data already contains sensitive and personal information. A prominent example of such data is medical and health data, which contains very sensitive patient information.

In this chapter, we will discuss how privacy of such data can be preserved without hindering the advances AI promises in this domain. We will discuss several solutions and provide use cases related to healthcare. While AI is being used to advance and automate many aspects and functions within healthcare, in this chapter, we constrain our discussion on addressing the privacy challenges posed by the need for health data to fuel AI-based healthcare algorithms. Such algorithms aim to improve medical practices, such as disease classification, disease detection, epidemic prediction and treatment plans. Discussion about AI operational advances in healthcare, such as those involving robotics (Pavel Hamet 2017), are excluded from the scope of this chapter.

## 2   AI in Healthcare

In healthcare, AI opens new doors for unprecedented opportunities that can advance medicine and solve long standing medical problems. With correct and adequate data, AI has the potential to lead for discoveries that can save lives. In particular, AI can provide data-driven Clinical Decision Support Systems (CDSS) that will optimize medical decisions and recommendations based on patient data (Melton 2017). AI can find hidden correlations among symptoms and diseases, and help prevent them. AI can also provide useful insights into current treatment plans and suggest ways to improve them. AI can analyze thousands of medical images and flag early detection alerts with reasonable accuracy, saving many laborious hours of specialized practitioners. When given appropriate data, AI can even predict disease outbreak and prevent epidemics.

However, all these potential advances are surrounded by privacy concerns because they are all being fueled by the same source: medical and health data. In one hand, for AI to advance state of the art, it needs access to data. In the other hand, privacy of patients whose data is being used by AI could easily be breached. In the following sections, we will discuss a few potential approaches and solutions that can elevate this dilemma.

# 3 Preserving Privacy

Advances in healthcare has led to a state of affairs where medical equipment are constantly generating extremely large volume of digital data, giving rise to what is commonly known today as the *medical big data* (Lee and Yoon 2017). Such data exhibits high degree of complexity and proved to be quite difficult to mine and analyze. At the same time, this data may well hold extremely valuable insights that can be used to advance healthcare, such as predicting epidemics or supporting effective treatment decisions.

Interestingly, the existence of such data makes healthcare an attractive platform for a sub-field of AI called *machine learning*. Machine learning analyzes large datasets to build mathematical models capable of predicting, classifying and clustering data based on insights acquired while analyzing it. Machine learning has evidently become an extremely powerful tool that not only improves the quality of data analytics, but also potentially maximizes the utility of big data; for machine learning, more training data (usually) means more accurate results.

However, while providing an increasingly attractive venue to advance healthcare, machine learning can conceivably breach the privacy of patients whose data is being used to train its models. In other words, to improve the accuracy of machine learning algorithms, we need to provide more training data; in healthcare, such data often includes very sensitive patient information. Therefore, the challenge is: how can we train machine learning algorithms with sufficient amount of data without exposing sensitive information? To answer this question, new directions of research have emerged attempting to achieve what is commonly known as *privacy-preserving machine learning*, or more generally *privacy-preserving AI*.

In the remaining of this section, we will discuss and illustrate the most common approaches to achieve privacy-preserving machine learning in general, while relating to use cases and applications in healthcare. Table 1 provides a comparison between the privacy-preserving approaches discussed in this chapter.

**Table 1** Privacy-preserving approaches

| Approach | Computation efficiency | Communication overhead | Privacy |
|---|---|---|---|
| Homomorphic encryption | Slow | Light | High |
| Multi-party computation | Moderate | High | High |
| Differential privacy | Moderate | Moderate | Moderate |
| Federated learning | Fast | Light | High |

## *3.1 Homomorphic Encryption*

The most straightforward solution to preserve privacy is to cryptographically protect the data, it is also usually the most inefficient. The standard scenario when operating on encrypted data is to decrypt it, perform the required computations then encrypt it again. Clearly, in this case, the privacy of data can be breached during the computation phase. Homomorphic encryption provides a solution. It *magically* allows operations to be computed over encrypted data to yield encrypted results, which, if decrypted by the same key that was used to encrypt it in the first place, would match the result of the required computation as if it was performed on the plain (un-encrypted) data.

Homomorphic Encryption can indeed preserve the privacy of patient data in many scenarios, such as when a particular healthcare organization intends to privately out-source machine learning computation on its data or when several healthcare entities decide to collaborate on a machine learning computation without having to expose their data to each other.

It might be hard to believe that such schemes are even possible, but let's consider an over-simplified example to illustrate the basic idea (Hayes 2012). Suppose that our encryption scheme is taking the logarithm of the data, hence the encryption of $x$ is $log(x)$. Now, suppose that we want to perform multiplication over positive integer numbers. Given the fact that $x \times y = z$ is equivalent to $log(x) + log(y) = log(z)$, a simple homomorphic encryption algorithm $E$ proceeds as follows:

1. Encrypt the values $x$ and $y$, such that $E(x) = log(x)$ and $E(y) = log(y)$.
2. Send $log(x)$ and $log(y)$ to an untrusted party, which performs basic addition $log(x) + log(y) = log(z)$
3. Obtain the result $log(z)$ and decrypt it by taking the anti-log. This will yield $z = x \times y$.

In the above example, the task was to multiply two numbers without revealing their values. Therefore, we encrypted the numbers, added the encrypted numbers, generated an encrypted result, and finally decrypted it to obtain the correct result, based on the fact that addition of encrypted values lead to multiplication of their corresponding plain values on that particular encryption scheme. Any party other than the owner of the data will not be able to find out what the results are, unless they can decrypt the data (i.e. possess knowledge of the key, which is, in this example, anti-log). In reality, encryption schemes are much more complex than merely taking logarithm of encryption and ani-logarithm for decryption.

In 2009, Gantry (2009) presented the first Fully Homomorphic Encryption scheme, which is the strongest Homomorphic Encryption notion that allows all operations (i.e. addition, multiplication, subtraction and division) unrestrictedly on encrypted data. Other types, which allow only some operations include Partially Homomorphic Encryption (Rivest et al. 1978), Somewhat Homomorphic Encryption (van Dijk et al. 2010), and Leveled Fully Homomorphic encryption (Brakerski et al. 2011). Recent advances offered many improvements to this class of schemes (Gentry et al. 2013; Brakerski and Vaikuntanathan 2014; Chillotti et al. 2016; Gama et al. 2016), and today there is a number of open source libraries for fully homomorphic encryption implementations, e.g.: HElib (Halevi and Shoup 2019), SEAL (2019), TFHE (Chillotti et al. 2016), PALISADE (2017), HEAAN (Cheon et al. 2017).

An example of privacy-preserving machine learning application in healthcare based on homomorphic encryption is presented in Vizitiu et al. (2019), where Homomorphic Encryption was used in medical imaging. It was shown that data encrypted with fully homomorphic encryption was used to classify X-Ray coronary angiography views with 96.2% accuracy.

However, while it is considered the most secure privacy-preserving approach, it is still (at the time of writing) very slow and not practically applicable for large datasets.

## 3.2  Multi-party Computation

In some scenarios, data are being shared between multiple parties, who are interested in leveraging their own data to improve some joint analysis, as it is often the case that analysis on larger datasets can yield results with better accuracy and more insights than those conducted on smaller dispersed datasets. However, will such parties be willing to share their data in plain? In most cases, unless the privacy of the shared data can be guaranteed, parties will not be willing to share their data.

One way to preserve the privacy of such data is through Multi-Party Computation (MPC) (Yao 1982). Basically, MPC is a protocol that enables a number of parties to provide inputs and collaboratively compute a value without actually revealing their inputs to each other. The basic idea is simple, each party splits their data and exchange the splits with other parties. Each party then performs the required computations on the splits and exchange them again. Finally, each party combine all the exchanged splits to reveal the result. MPC guarantees that the result is correct as if the computation has been performed on the plain data. Operations such as addition and multiplication can be computed efficiently, but others such as comparison, are slightly more complex. This approach is called MPC based on *secret sharing*. The most popular MPC protocol based on secret sharing is SPDZ (Damgård 2012), which is implemented in the library SCALE-MAMBA (KU Leuven: SCALE-MAMBA 2019).

In healthcare, such scenario is commonplace. For example, suppose that Hospital A possesses data about patients that have been diagnosed with disease D. Hospital A performed some analysis on its data and obtained results, but thinks that the accuracy can be improved if data from other hospitals (Hospital B and Hospital C) about the same disease D are used to complement its own data. Hospital B and Hospital C would, of course, be very reluctant to share their data, but at the same time believe that they too would benefit from having access to the data of Hospital A. In this case, MPC provides a solution that allows Hospitals A, B and C to collaboratively and privately compute the required result. Suppose that the information hospitals are interested in is calculating the total number of cases that have been diagnosed with disease D across the three hospitals. Assuming that the total number of cases in Hospital A, Hospital B and Hospital C, are $X, Y, Z$, respectively, a simple MPC protocol proceeds as follows:

1. Hospital A splits $X$ to $x_1 + x_2$
2. Hospital B splits $Y$ to $y_1 + y_2$
3. Hospital C splits $Z$ to $z_1 + z_2$
4. Hospital A sends $x_2$ to Hospital B
5. Hospital B sends $y_2$ to Hospital C
6. Hospital C sends $z_2$ to Hospital A
7. Hospital A calculates the sum of all its splits: $x_1 + z_2 = A_{share}$
8. Hospital B calculates the sum of all its splits: $y_1 + x_2 = B_{share}$
9. Hospital B calculates the sum of all its splits: $z_1 + y_2 = C_{share}$

The total number of cases can easily be obtained by $A_{share} + B_{share} + C_{share}$ without knowing what the values of $X, Y, Z$ were. That is

$$A_{share} + B_{share} + C_{share} = (x_1 + z_2) + (y_1 + x_2) + (z_1 + y_2)$$

rearranging the terms, we have

$$(x_1 + x_2) + (y_1 + y_2) + (z_1 + z_2) = X + Y + Z$$

Fig. 1 illustrates this example.

A practical application of the use of MPC in healthcare is presented in Jagadeesh et al. (2017) for genomatic diseases, where the authors were able to discover previously unrecognized disease genes, while preserving the privacy of the participating patients through MPC.

While it still suffers from degraded efficiency, MPC is order of magnitude more efficient than Homomorphic Encryption. However, MPC introduces communication

**Fig. 1** Multi-party computation

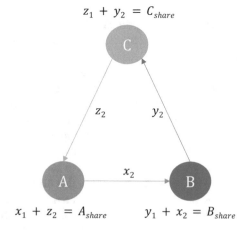

overhead due the high volume of interactions among the parties during computation; this makes MPC suitable only for small number of collaborating parties.

## 3.3 Differential Privacy

Unlike Homomorphic Encryption and MPC, Differential Privacy (DP) (Dwork et al. 2006) is a more general and much faster approach, and it does not involve encrypting the data. The basic idea of DP is to add noise to the data before giving an external party access to it.

In a typical DP scenario, a computing party (a party that would like to perform some computation over external data) queries a data owner. The data owner then adds some noise to the response before sending it to the computing party, such noise should hide the actual data (preserve privacy) while allowing the computing party to correctly carry out the required computation. However, DP is a trade-off between privacy and accuracy, the more noise you add to the data, the better the privacy, but the lower the accuracy, and vice versa. This is captured in the notion of *privacy budget*, which dictates how many queries are allowed and how much noise can be added to the data to maintain the balance between privacy and accuracy (high budge implies more queries, which, in turn, may result in less privacy). A remarkable work in this area is the the PATE framework (Papernot et al. 2016), which not only maintains the noise budget regardless of the number of the queries, but also improves both learning and privacy.

DP can be conducted based on two approaches, either local DP or Global DP. In local DP, the data owners add noise to their data and send it to an aggregator, which, as its name suggests, aggregates the (noisy) data and sends it to the computing party (which typically runs some machine learning algorithm). This approach can become extremely noisy as the number of data owners grow. In this case, the global DP is more desirable, where the data owners trust the aggregator and send their data without noise, then it is the responsibility of the aggregator to aggregate and add noise to the data before forwarding it to the computing party. Figure 2 illustrates both local and global DP.

In healthcare, DP has been extensively used (Moussa and Demurjian 2017). An example of a practical application of DP in healthcare is cohort identification (Vinterbo et al. 2012). In this scenario, a database holding patient information is queried for suitable subjects to be recruited for some clinical trails.

DP is the preferred approached when a large volume of data needs to be processed (in which case, Homomorphic Encryption and MPC would be much slower options). DP is a practical solution and is in fact already being used on products by major industry vendors, such as Apple and Google, to privately collect data from their customers.

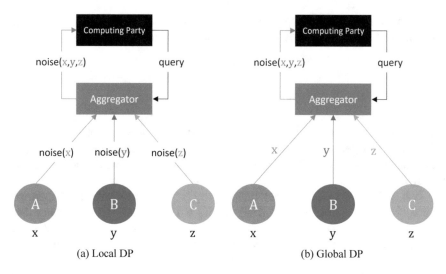

**Fig. 2** Differential privacy

## 3.4   Federated Learning

A more recent approach to address privacy concerns when sharing sensitive data is *Federated Learning*, which was proposed by Google in 2017 (Brendan McMahan et al. 2017). Federated learning is structurally similar to DP, with one big difference: in federated learning, the data never leaves the repositories of their owners. Instead of adding noise to the data before sending it off to be used to train a machine learning model externally, as the case in DP, in federated learning, the actual machine learning model is sent to the data owners, who perform the computation locally, improve the model and then send the improved model (i.e. the model's parameters) back to a central server. The improved models received from all participating data owners are then aggregated (e.g., averaged out) to produce a global optimal model, which is then sent to the participating nodes to update their local copies of the model; these iterations are called federated rounds. This process is repeated continuously until the maximum number of federated rounds is reached (which is set by the global server). Figure 3 illustrates the basic operation of typical federated learning process as described above.

Federated Learning effectively promotes a new approach of machine learning, one where the training of data takes place in a decentralized manner. In addition to privacy, such approach offers other attractive benefits:

- distributed computation: computation is performed by many nodes rather than a central one
- distributed storage: data is not stored in a central location
- lower network cost: only the parameters of the model are transmitted rather than the actual data.

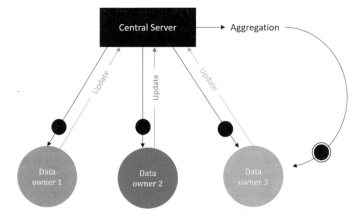

**Fig. 3** Federated learning

An example of a recent healthcare application utilizing federated learning is presented in Brisimi et al. (2018), where a machine learning algorithm is proposed to predict hospitalization due to heart disease by analyzing their health records in a decentralized fashion.

Popular frameworks and open libraries such as TensorFlow by Google and PyTorch by Facebook have already incorporated federated learning. However, federated learning is still in its infancy and more effort is required to formalize its potential (that is in contrast with DP, which is generally more understood and has solid theoretical foundation).

In healthcare, federated learning promises a lot of potential and seem to offer balanced solutions for common data privacy concerns. Furthermore, under some legislation, data is prohibited to leave a particular geographical location, even if it was anonymous or scumbled. In such cases, federated learning might be the only option to enable optimal learning on scale.

## 4 Legal Framework

Health data is often believed to be fully legally protected by well-established legislations, such as the Health Insurance Portability and Accountability Act of 1996 (HIPAA) in the United State, which provides privacy and security for medical records. However, does HIPAA also cover the emerging privacy concerns due to AI? Recent study refutes (Kulkarni 2019).

One approach to use healthcare data while still preserving its privacy is to anonymize it by removing any personal identification data that may identify the subjects (i.e. patients). However, it turns out it is not difficult to de-anonymize the data using standard machine learning algorithms. Recent research (Na et al. 2018) demonstrated that using large anonymized national physical activity dataset, it was possible to de-anonymize the subjects whose data belong to citizens only by aggregating some demographic information such as, age, sex, race/ethnicity and education level. While the requirement of using demographic information (which might not always be available) limit the accuracy of such approach, the fact that it was possible at the first place, even with access to these demographic information, is quite alarming and does trigger an urgent call to review the current anonymization techniques.

HIPAA was originally provisioned to protect health data assuming it resides at healthcare organizations. However, once health data leaves healthcare organization, it is no longer covered by HIPAA. The pervasiveness of technology today resulted on decentralized measurement and storage of health data. In the past, healthcare organizations were probably the only place where collecting health data is possible, basically because they were the only place with equipment capable of taking health measurements. Today, this is not the case. With advances in consumer technologies, even wearable devices can now take very detailed and thorough measurements about individuals and generate reasonably accurate health data. This effectively brings technology companies into the scope as they collect health data about their customers, sometimes without their consent. Even worse, in these situations, there is no clear regulation on how such data should be stored, protected and used.

However, in May 2018, the world witnessed a milestone in privacy protection legislation, this time it was from Europe. GDPR (General Data Protection Regulation) is a European legislation that regulates how data belonging to EU citizens should be collected, processed and stored; unlike HIPAA, GPDR covers all industries handling such data, not just healthcare organizations. In fact, any organization handling EU citizens data should comply with GDPR, even if it was physically located and operating outside the EU. GPDR gives citizens more control over the data that is being collected about them and more visibility on how it is being used. GDPR further explicitly defines the individual's rights over their data. For example, GDPR defines the Right To Be Forgotten (RTBF), which gives the individual the right to request permanent erasure of their data, and the right for correction, which gives the individual the right to correct their data.

Healthcare was probably the industry affected the most by the new law, where GDPR was seen both as an opportunity and a challenge. Fully complying with GDPR, at least for healthcare, meant a revamp of how patient data is handled, especially for organizations that are not already HIPAA compliant. At the same time, GDPR became an opportunity to standardize and improve data management policies within healthcare; a long journey that has just started.

## 5   Concluding Remarks

We should carefully manage data and preserve its privacy as we are harnessing the potential AI can bring to healthcare. In this chapter, we illustrated how AI can conceivably breach the privacy of data when deployed in healthcare organizations.

We then discussed how recent advances in technology provided some solutions. In particular, we discussed four such solutions: homomorphic encryption, multi-party computation, differential privacy and federated learning. We discussed these solutions in detail and gave applications related to healthcare, while presenting both their promises and drawbacks. Depending on the application, some of these solutions may be more suitable than others; it is, therefore, very important that context is well understood before adopting any of these solutions.

Finally, we discussed the issue of heath data privacy from legal prospective, and showed that while conventional healthcare legislation, such as HIPAA of the United States, may not cover recent applications involving health data, GDPR of the European Union has remarkably treated data privacy issues in greater depth while covering modern applications.

Looking ahead, we will likely see transformative attempts to address data privacy in healthcare. Once such attempt has recently been trending, namely, using blockchain in healthcare (Mettler 2016), which introduces a new approach, where data is managed and protected in a decentralized manner. While blockchain has steeply hyped on several industries over the past few years as a futuristic promising technology, its true potential is still not very well understood and has indeed initiated some arguments that will likely last for a few years to come.

# References

Brakerski Z, Gentry C, Vaikuntanathan V (2011) (Leveled) fully homomorphic encryption without bootstrapping. Electron Colloquium Comput Complexity. https://doi.org/10.1145/2090236. 2090262

Brakerski Z, Vaikuntanathan V (2014) Lattice-based FHE as secure as PKE. In: Proceedings of the 5th conference on innovations in theoretical computer science. https://doi.org/10.1145/2554797. 2554799

Brendan McMahan H, Moore E, Ramage D, Hampson S, Arcas B (2017) Communication-efficient learning of deep networks from decentralized data. Artif Intell Stat

Brisimi T, Chen R, Mela T, Olshevsky A, Paschalidis I, Shi W (2018) Federated learning of predictive models from federated electronic health records. Int J Med Inform 112:59–67 ISSN: 1872-8243. https://doi.org/10.1016/j.ijmedinf.2018.01.007

Cheon JH, Kim A, Kim M, Song Y (2017) Homomorphic encryption for arithmetic of approximate numbers. In: Takagi T, Peyrin T (eds) Advances in cryptology—ASIACRYPT 2017. ASIACRYPT 2017. Springer, Cham, pp 409–437. https://doi.org/10.1007/978-3-319-70694-8_15

Chillotti I, Gama N, Georgieva M, Izabachène M (2016) Faster fully homomorphic encryption: bootstrapping in less than 0.1 seconds. In: Cheon J, Takagi T (eds) Advances in cryptology—ASIACRYPT 2016. ASIACRYPT 2016. Lecture notes in computer science, vol 10031. Springer, Berlin. https://doi.org/10.1007/978-3-662-53887-6_1

Chillotti I,Gama N, Georgieva M, Izabachène M (2016) TFHE: fast fully homomorphic encryption library. https://tfhe.github.io/tfhe/

Damgård I, Pastro V, Smart N, Zakarias S (2012) Multiparty computation from somewhat homomorphic encryption. In: Safavi-Naini R, Canetti R (eds) Advances in cryptology—CRYPTO 2012. CRYPTO 2012. Lecture notes in computer science, vol 7417. Springer, Berlin. https://doi.org/10.1007/978-3-642-32009-5_38

Dwork C, McSherry F, Nissim K, Smith A (2006) Calibrating noise to sensitivity in private data analysis. In: Halevi S, Rabin T (eds) Proceedings of the third conference on theory of cryptography (TCC'06). Springer, Berlin, pp 265–284. https://doi.org/10.1007/11681878_14

Gama N, Izabachène M, Nguyen PQ, Xie X (2016) Structural lattice reduction: generalized worst-case to average-case reductions and homomorphic cryptosystems. In: Fischlin M, Coron JS (eds) Advances in cryptology—EUROCRYPT 2016. EUROCRYPT 2016. Lecture notes in computer science, vol 9666. Springer, Berlin. https://doi.org/10.1007/978-3-662-49896-5_19

Gentry C (2009) Fully homomorphic encryption using ideal lattices. In: the 41st ACM symposium on theory of computing. https://doi.org/10.1145/1536414.1536440

Gentry C, Sahai A, Waters B (2013) Homomorphic encryption from learning with errors: conceptually-simpler, asymptotically-faster, attribute-based. In: Canetti R, Garay JA (eds) Advances in cryptology—CRYPTO 2013. CRYPTO 2013. Lecture notes in computer science, vol 8042. Springer, Berlin. https://doi.org/10.1007/978-3-642-40041-4_5

Halevi S, Shoup V (2019) HElib: An Implementation of homomorphic encryption. https://github.com/homenc/HElib. Cited Nov 2019

Hayes B (2012) Alice and Bob in cipherspace. Am Scientist. https://doi.org/10.1511/2012.98.362

Jagadeesh K, Wu D, Birgmeierm J, Boneh D, Bejerano G (2017) Deriving genomic diagnoses without revealing patient genomes. Science 357(6352):692–695. https://doi.org/10.1126/science.aam9710

KU Leuven: SCALE-MAMBA. https://homes.esat.kuleuven.be/~nsmart/SCALE. Cited Nov 2019

Kulkarni A (2019) AI in healthcare: data privacy and ethics concerns. https://www.lexalytics.com/lexablog/ai-healthcare-data-privacy-ethics-issues. Cited Nov 2019

Lee CH, Yoon HJ (2017) Medical big data: promise and challenges. Kidney Res Clin Pract. https://doi.org/10.23876/j.krcp.2017.36.1.3

Melton BL (2017) Systematic review of medical informatics-supported medication decision making. Biomed Inform Insights. https://doi.org/10.1177/1178222617697975

Mettler M (2016) Blockchain technology in healthcare: the revolution starts here. In: IEEE 18th international conference on e-health networking, applications and services. https://doi.org/10.1109/HealthCom.2016.7749510

Microsoft research: Microsoft SEAL. https://www.microsoft.com/en-us/research/project/microsoft-seal. Cited Nov 2019

Moussa M, Demurjian S (2017) Differential privacy approach for big data privacy in healthcare. In: Tamane S, Solanki VK, Dey N (eds) Privacy and security policies in big data. IGI Global, pp 191–213. https://doi.org/10.4018/978-1-5225-2486-1.ch009

Na L, Yang C, Lo C, Zhao F, Fukuoka Y, Aswani A (2018) Feasibility of reidentifying individuals in large national physical activity data sets from which protected health information has been removed with use of machine learning. JAMA Netw Open. https://doi.org/10.1001/jamanetworkopen.2018.6040

Palisade Homomorphic Encryption Software Library (2017). https://palisade-crypto.org/

Papernot N, Abadi M, Erlingsson U, Goodfellow I, Talwar K (2016) Semi-supervised knowledge transfer for deep learning from private training data. https://arxiv.org/abs/1610.05755. Cited Nov 2019

Pavel Hamet P, Tremblay J (2017) Artificial intelligence in medicine. Metabolism. https://doi.org/10.1016/j.metabol.2017.01.011

Rivest R, Shamir A, Adleman L (1978) A method for obtaining digital signatures and public-key cryptosystems. Commun ACM. https://doi.org/10.1145/359340.359342

van Dijk M, Gentry C, Halevi S, Vaikuntanathan V (2010) Fully homomorphic encryption over the integers. In: Gilbert H (eds) Advances in cryptology—EUROCRYPT 2010. EUROCRYPT 2010. Lecture notes in computer science, vol 6110. Springer, Berlin. https://doi.org/10.1007/978-3-642-13190-5_2

Vinterbo S, Sarwate A, Boxwala A (2012) Protecting count queries in study design. J Am Med Inform Assoc. https://doi.org/10.1136/amiajnl-2011-000459

Vizitiu A, Niţă C, Puiu A, Suciu C, Itu L (2019) Towards privacy-preserving deep learning based medical imaging applications. In: IEEE international symposium on medical measurements and applications (MeMeA). Istanbul, Turkey, pp 1–6. https://doi.org/10.1109/MeMeA.2019.8802193

Yao A, Protocols for secure computations. In: Proceedings of the 23rd annual symposium on foundations of computer science (SFCS '82). IEEE Computer Society, Washington, DC, USA, pp 160–164. https://doi.org/10.1109/SFCS.1982.88

# Patients Perspective—Benefits and Challenges of Artificial Intelligence

**Usman Iqbal, Hafsah Arshed Ali Khan, and Yu-Chuan (Jack) Li**

**Abstract** Artificial Intelligence's implementation into medicine, research, and crisis management have changed the way healthcare are delivered to the population. The beneficial qualities of Artificial Intelligence in medicine are profound, but it is a field often subject to grandiloquent claims. Patient's perspective could be better and understood and their involvement in developing health technology software would prove greatly beneficial. As Taiwan's databases of medical information are growing, the cost of analyzing data is falling, and more and more professionals and investors are showing interest in being a part of this burgeoning phenomenon.

## 1 Artificial Intelligence: A Toolbox of Potential

As the once imagined future quickly becomes the present, technological advances are slowly becoming part and parcel of everyday life. Machine Intelligence, or more commonly, Artificial Intelligence (AI) is a branch of computer science involving machines and programs that can emulate critical thinking and decision-making skills similar to humans. Artificial Intelligence has made gathering, storing, organizing, and retrieving data extraordinarily efficient and is aiding in difficult decision making in various aspects of medical crisis. Studies have reviewed current applications of AI, as well as the opportunities and challenges it poses in the field of health care. To quote examples, severity scoring systems have utilized AI for some time now, and researchers are wondering if it can also be used to aid mental health workers in suicidal risk assessment or physicians in the screening of rare genetic conditions (Abazeed 2019).

U. Iqbal (✉) · H. Arshed Ali Khan · Y.-C. Li
International Center for Health Information Technology (ICHIT), Taipei Medical University, No. 172-1, Sec. 2, Keelung Rd., Daan District, Taipei City 106, Taiwan
e-mail: usmaniqbal@tmu.edu.tw

Y.-C. Li
e-mail: jack@tmu.edu.tw

© Springer Nature Switzerland AG 2021
M. Househ et al. (eds.), *Multiple Perspectives on Artificial Intelligence in Healthcare*,
Lecture Notes in Bioengineering, https://doi.org/10.1007/978-3-030-67303-1_7

## 2  Artificial Intelligence and Decision Making in Health Systems

The ever increasing burden of illness, aging driven disability, multiple morbidities, as well as increased demand and cost of healthcare services, are among some of the challenges faced by health systems worldwide (Panch et al. 2018).

Health care systems have a framework that constitutes the collection and processing of information. Policymakers must effectively manage these systems by adjusting the organization, governance, and handling of finance and resources to achieve efficiency, i.e. health system outputs (health care services and public health) and system goals.

The delivery of health care is primarily a multistep process. The core information processing tasks involved include screening and diagnosis as well as monitoring and treatment. Breaking things down further, the general method of managing these processes across the vast areas of health system management and healthcare delivery involves the generation and testing of the hypothesis and then action (implementation). AI can potentially, within a health system, better hypothesis generation, and testing by revealing previously obscure trends in data. This is substantial at all levels of the system.

There are some AI applications already in use, specifically in public health, affecting health providers and patients alike. Some programs provide adverse drug reaction and interaction warnings during the prescription of medicine, patient reminder calls for appointments, decision-support tools for clinicians, and robotic surgical systems.

An interesting point to note is that Artificial Intelligence, despite being primed to alter patient engagement in healthcare, the patient's perspective on the matter is poorly understood (Nelson et al. 2020).

## 3  Ethical Concerns Around Use of Artificial Intelligence

The concerns raised around the plans to implement Artificial Intelligence into such a vital part of human life are many. Policies and guidelines for the use of this technology do exist but are they keeping up with the ongoing progress and development in machine learning and its implementation in medicine? Medical staff are some people at the very forefront of this process and there are efforts to educate, update and engage the community in conversation regarding the ethical concerns of AI. However, the complex nature of this technology leaves room for further discussions (Rigby 2019).

It is important that AI approaches in medical practice is lawful, ethical, and robust. The Eruopean Union (EU) guidelines for trustworthy AI state seven critical requirements for ethical AI: human agency and oversight, technical reliability and safety; privacy and data governance; transparency; diversity, non-discrimination, and fairness; societal and environmental wellbeing; and accountability (Kazim and

Koshiyama 2020). This includes tiered, risk-based guidance for tool validation for prevention of harm, recommendations to make the model understandable as well as fair and unbiased, and ensuring that human autonomy is preserved. In accordance with the guidelines, the implementation of AI should enhance and build upon the actions of humans through pathways that are transparent and traceable rather than black-box decision making.

An AI model is in a state of constant evolution. The matter to consider is how these inevitable changes to AI models should be regulated after they are granted approval for use in the clinic. This is addressed by the US Food and Drug Administration (FDA) whitepaper on modifications to software using machine learning models (FDA 2019) These are not formal guidelines yet; however, the framework that has been issued for discussion is thought-provoking and identifies the three main areas under which the AI can evolve: performance, input, and the software's intended use. The latter could be grounds for restarting the approval procedure, whereas other adjustments need only be recorded and subjected to periodical review (Tran et al. 2019).

## 4 Patient Perspectives About AI and Associated Health Technologies

It is without a doubt that humans and technologies can bring forth a new era of efficiency, achieving goals with higher proficiency in half the time. This collaboration has the potential to tackle many, if not most of the vulnerabilities of the current system.

There are many misconceptions and lack of complete information available to most in regards to AI in medicine and health care technologies. Will machine replace physicians? Does software have the ability to comprehend difficult lifestyles and situations and display empathy? Will the integrity of the physician–patient relationship be compromised and how transparent is the use of a patient's health data? Can AI make mistakes and if yes, what then?

Artificial Intelligence provides the exponential enhancement to human-driven science in gathering, filtering and organizing data. However, as in many ways, Artificial Intelligence and Health Technologies are still in their infancy, understanding the comprehension of the patients (the owners of this data) is pivotal in further developing the system to unlock its full potential. Patients' knowledge and awareness of Artificial Intelligence and the resulting technologies is mostly from mass media, educational events and some personal encounters.

Artificial Intelligence is set to alter the way patients access health care however, there is much to learn about the patient perspectives on the matter. (Nelson et al. 2020) People play a major role in their own health care being able to decide when, how and where to seek help in case of an illness or trauma. It is then vital that they know enough and fully comprehend their situation to be able to make sound decisions regarding the health care they will receive. (Cosgriff and Celi 2020).

The online symptom checker system's accuracy is an ongoing concern in the general community; however a major group of patient-users find an AI-assisted program such as this very useful. Formal validation studies gauging the symptom checker precision and efficacy in real-world practice could provide added useful insight into their value (Meyer et al. 2020).

A qualitative study conducted in dermatology assessed the potential for direct-to-patient and clinician decision-support AI tools in order to categorize lesions of the skin. This study showed that patients were receptive to the utilization of Artificial Intelligence for the screening of skin cancer if it can be done without sacrificing the integrity of the human physician–patient connection (Nelson et al. 2020). Another example is the wearable biometric monitoring devices (BMDs) coupled with AI that allow for the remote measurement and the analysis of patient data in real time. The data point collected from these devices are in the thousands and can assist in diagnosis, predicting outcomes and aiding health professionals pick the best treatment plan individually tailored to their patients. The reception to these devices has been favorable, however without the information on their usefulness to a patient its hard to comment on their effectiveness.

Another study found that in general, patients are not very optimistic about AI-based systems replacing radiologists in diagnostic interpretations. The patient wanted to be kept in the loop regarding every step of the diagnostic process. They also expressed the need for human interaction in the case of communicating the results. This study concluded that it is vital to involve patients in the development of Artificial Intelligence-based systems and technologies that deal with diagnosis, management, and prognosis as well as the development of ethical and legal frameworks within which these systems are allowed to operate (Ongena et al. 2019).

So far, Artificial Intelligence can only be developed for challenges that are already completely understood. It does not seem like human supervision would not be required for the operation of these systems to smooth out or make up for any flaws or possible deficits. AI is a tool to enhance and better the existing medical system in addition to its existing components. There are multiple bodies producing guidelines for the safe, trustworthy development of AI (Lennon et al. 2017). EU guidelines, promote the development of trustworthy AI across all disciplines, a US Food and Drug Administration whitepaper proposes a regulatory framework for constantly developing software in health care. Guidelines from the National Institution of Health and Care Excellence (NICE) handle the level of evidence required for new digital health intervention, and NHSX and Public Health England have reported intentions to produce their own AI guidelines (Abazeed 2019). This effort, coupled with data transparency, maintenance of physician–patient confidentiality and constant patient education and feedback, could potentially usher in the new age of health care, with Artificial Intelligence, Big Data and technology to aid us in our day to day lives as well as time of health crisis.

## 5  Taiwan's Health Technology Journey and Initiatives in Global Crisis

Taiwan's single-payer system successfully implemented adoption of Health Information Technology (HIT) on a national scale; from flash drive to health cloud and big data to open data (Iqbal et al. 2017; Li et al. 2018). Taiwan's innovative history within the health technology arena has made it a strategic contender in the global marathon of innovations. Local and international multidisciplinary collaboration has been critical to this ongoing success whilst the hackathon model has been imperative in fostering the required alliance. We hope that through events we can begin to address not only the technical issues that surround health, but the additional barriers of cost, accessibility and usability. It is certainly a time of great growth and excitement surrounding Health technology innovations and only through collaborative work can we hope to reach its full potential (Iqbal et al. 2018).

The Health Information Technology advancements has expedited the gathering of observational health data in Taiwan and worldwide. This is easily reflected in the universal coverage of the 23 million Taiwanese populace with the hundred percent e-claims and very accessible clinics and hospitals (Li et al. 2015). The National Health Insurance Research Database (NHIRD) was established by the NHI 20 years ago. This system gathers information on patient visits from all over Taiwan (Fig. 1) This

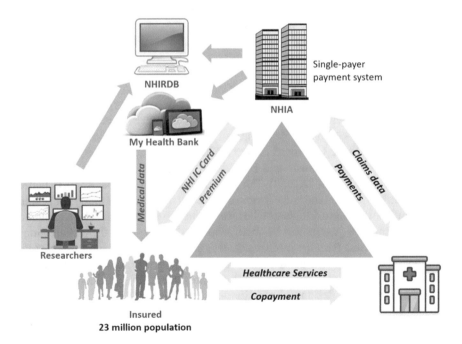

**Fig. 1**  Taiwan's national health insurance administration structure

extensive, detailed, specific data gathered by the cumulative healthcare body is the cornerstone of clinical research and healthcare (Hsing and Ioannidis 2015).

Following the SARS outbreak in 2003, Taiwan established a public health response system in preparation for another potential crisis. During the recent COVID19 (Novel Coronavirus) pandemic, teams of officials were well-prepared to promptly launch into action (Wang et al. 2020). While the outbreak was still in its infancy, Taiwan leveraged its national health insurance database and integrated it with its immigration and customs database to initiate the construction of big data for analytics. If an individual visited a clinic or hospital, that data would generate alerts based on the patient's symptoms and travel history. At the nation's borders, those considered low risk were sent a pass via text message allowing them entry. Anyone considered high risk was put into self-isolation and monitored through their mobile phone to ensure that they remained at home during the quarantine period. Given the continuing global spread of the disease, studying Taiwan's quick response and the management of disease outcomes may be beneficial for other countries.

## 6   MyHealthbank—eMask Initiative

In 2014, the NHI Administration established the official website for the MyHealth-Bank system. The main purpose of MyHealthBank is to provide NHI insured with their personal health-related information, to give right accessing their health care information, and to empower them for manage their own health. MyHealthBank contains AI based risk prediction models for certain disease like liver cancer however, needed further (Iqbal et al. 2017; Li et al. 2018).

During the COVID19 Health crisis, the eMask facility was introduced. This feature allowed people to purchase facemasks online instead of having to crowd Pharmacies and exposing themselves to potential illness. This initiative was well-received by the populace. Due to high demand, name-based rationing was applied to masks. The Central Epidemic Command Center (CECC) announced on March 2020 that an online ordering mechanism will be added to the name-based rationing system for face masks on March 12, 2020. The purpose of this new mechanism is to better ensure even distribution and make it more convenient to obtain face masks for people such as office workers and students who lack the time to go to pharmacies and public health centers. The government has been working tirelessly with the private sector to develop and test the new mechanism, which serves as an addition to existing distribution channels, i.e., pharmacies contracted by the Taiwan National Health Insurance Administration and local public health centers. The mechanism allowed people to order at a designated website using their NHI card or Citizen Digital Certificate or through the NHI app ("National Health Insurance Administration, Ministry of Health and Welfare, Taiwan (ROC)" 2020).

The CECC ran the first round of online orders beginning on March 12, 2020 and constituted a trial run, with an estimated seven million face masks (equal to the weekly allotment of 2.33 million people) being made available ("National Health

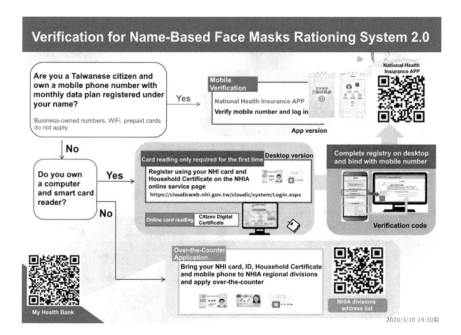

**Fig. 2** Verification ways for name-based mask reservation via MyhealthBank

Insurance Administration, Ministry of Health and Welfare, Taiwan (ROC)" 2020). By just opening the NHI APP and click "My Health Bank", users can easily start to make masks reservation using their mobile phone as shown in Figs. 2, 3 and 4 respectively ("National Health Insurance Administration, Ministry of Health and Welfare, Taiwan (ROC)" 2020). Though eMask is not directly based on AI model but this feature or similar could be enhanced in future to control infections by developing AI based smart monitoring and surveillance systems.

# 7 Conclusion

In the age of Big Data and Health Information Technology, Artificial Intelligence has the potential to speed up data gathering using health applications/health data banks and biometric monitoring devices as well as filter and categorize them efficiently. This will increase the efficiency and accuracy of diagnosis, treatment plans, prognosis as well as clinical research and crisis response. Patient's perspective could be better and understood and their involvement in developing health technology software would prove greatly beneficial.

The government of Taiwan had the 2003 SARS outbreak for reference and has established a public health response mechanism, enabling rapid actions for the next crisis. Well-trained and experienced teams of officials were quick to recognize the

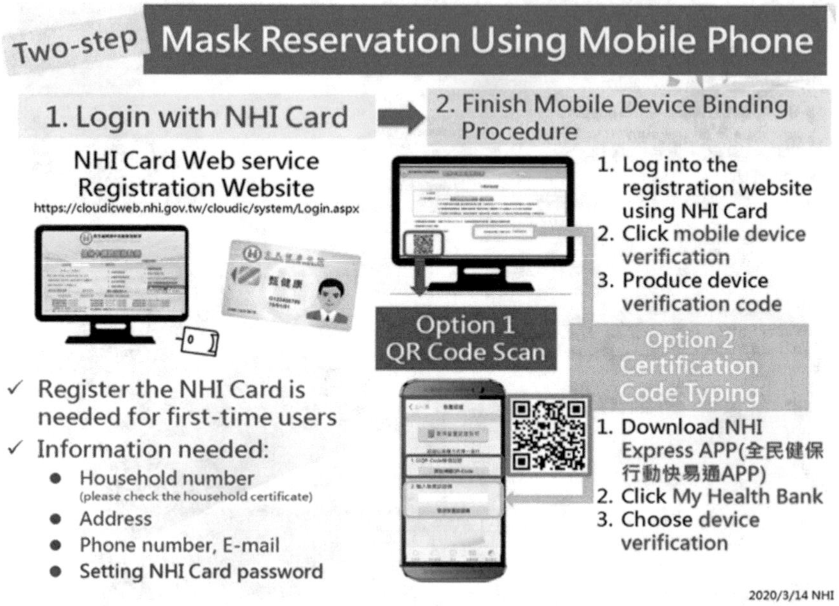

**Fig. 3** National health insurance express MobileApp verification steps guidance

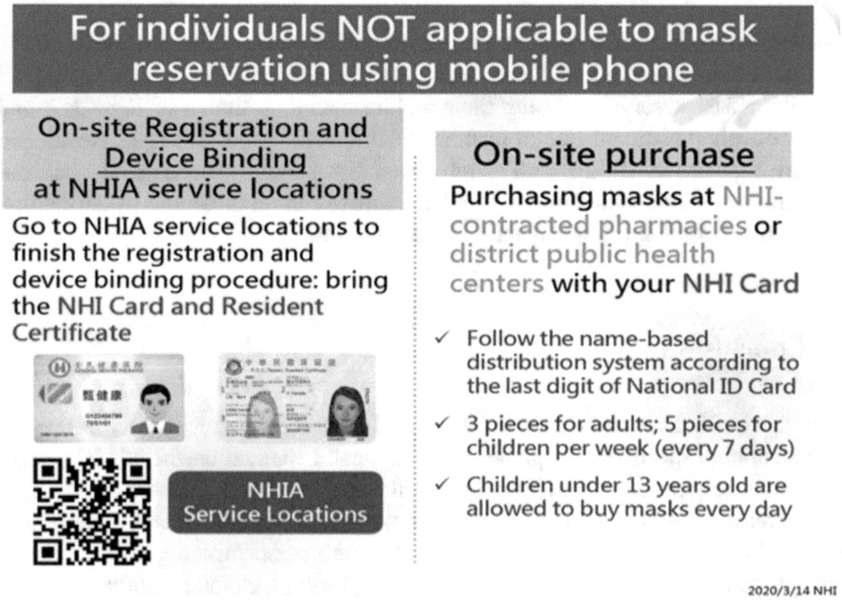

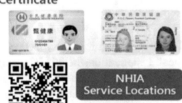

**Fig. 4** Guidance steps for individuals not applicable to reserve masks using mobile phones

crisis and activated emergency management structures to address the emerging outbreak. Taiwan's HIT journey from flash drive to Health Cloud showing the achievements of Taiwanese government in taking successful steps for health IT strategies development with time. Taiwan leveraged its national health insurance database and integrated it with its immigration and customs database to begin the creation of big data for analytics and controlled the health crisis COVID19.

The primary purpose of these initiatives is to ensure safety, sustain the continuity of care by providing patients information at the point of care regardless of where they get care, and to improve the quality of care. The meaningful use of Taiwan's MyHealthBank was also seen in the COVID19 Health crisis, where the Taiwanese government introduced the eMask facility that allows citizens to order online Facemasks instead going to the Pharmacy and be in queue for hours.

# References

Abazeed ME (2019) Walking the tightrope of artificial intelligence guidelines in clinical practice

Cosgriff CV, Celi LA (2020) Exploiting temporal relationships in the prediction of mortality. The Lancet Digital Health

FDA U (2019) Proposed regulatory framework for modifications to artificial intelligence/machine learning (AI/ML)-based software as a medical device (SaMD). In: FDA

Hsing AW, Ioannidis JPA (2015) Nationwide population science: lessons from the Taiwan national health insurance research database. JAMA Intern Med 175(9):1527–1529. https://doi.org/10.1001/jamainternmed.2015.3540

Iqbal U, Dagan A, Syed-Abdul S, Celi LA, Malwade S, Hsu MH, Li YJ (2018) A hackathon promoting Taiwanese health-IoT innovation. Comput Methods Programs Biomed 163:29–32. https://doi.org/10.1016/j.cmpb.2018.05.020

Iqbal U, Li Y-C, Lee WC, Hsu MH (2017) Taiwan's health information technology journey: from flash drive to health cloud. In: Health systems improvement across the globe: success stories from 60 countries

Kazim E, Koshiyama A (2020) Lack of vision: a comment on the EU's white paper on artificial intelligence. Available at SSRN 3558279

Lennon MR, Bouamrane M-M, Devlin AM, O'Connor S, O'Donnell C, Chetty U, Finch T (2017) Readiness for delivering digital health at scale: lessons from a longitudinal qualitative evaluation of a national digital health innovation program in the United Kingdom. J Med Internet Res 19(2):e42

Li Y-C et al. (2015) Building a national electronic medical record exchange system – experiences in Taiwan. Comput Methods Programs Biomed 121(1):14–20. https://doi.org/10.1016/j.cmpb.2015.04.013

Li Y-CJ, Lee W-C, Hsu M-HM, Iqbal U (2018) Taiwan: "my data, my decision": Taiwan's health improvement journey from big data to open data. In: Healthcare systems, pp 433–442. CRC Press

Meyer AN, Giardina TD, Spitzmueller C, Shahid U, Scott TM, Singh H (2020) Patient perspectives on the usefulness of an artificial intelligence-assisted symptom checker: cross-sectional survey study. J Med Internet Res 22(1):e14679

National Health Insurance Administration, Ministry of Health and Welfare, Taiwan (ROC) (2020) Retrieved from https://www.nhi.gov.tw/english/Content_List.aspx?n=022B9D97EF66C076

Nelson CA, Pérez-Chada LM, Creadore A, Li SJ, Lo K, Manjaly P, Mostaghimi A (2020) Patient perspectives on the use of artificial intelligence for skin cancer screening: a qualitative study. JAMA Dermatol. https://doi.org/10.1001/jamadermatol.2019.5014

Ongena YP, Haan M, Yakar D, Kwee TC (2019) Patients' views on the implementation of artificial intelligence in radiology: development and validation of a standardized questionnaire. European Radiol 1–8

Panch T, Szolovits P, Atun R (2018) Artificial intelligence, machine learning and health systems. J Global Health 8(2)

Rigby MJ (2019) Ethical dimensions of using artificial intelligence in health care. AMA J Ethics 21(2):121–124

Tran V-T, Riveros C, Ravaud P (2019) Patients' views of wearable devices and AI in healthcare: findings from the ComPaRe e-cohort. npj Digital Med 2(1):53. https://doi.org/10.1038/s41746-019-0132-y

Wang CJ, Ng CY, Brook RH (2020) Response to COVID-19 in Taiwan: Big data analytics, new technology, and proactive testing. JAMA. https://doi.org/10.1001/jama.2020.3151

# AI From a Health Professional Perspective

# Artificial Intelligence and Medication Management

Aude Motulsky, Jean-Noel Nikiema, and Delphine Bosson-Rieutort

**Abstract** Artificial intelligence in general, and machine learning (ML) techniques in particular, hold the promise of enormous benefits to medication management, both in the hospital or in the community setting. The potential of ML techniques to support the decision making of patients, clinicians, managers and/or policy-makers is massive. However, the learning will only be as good as the data, and the frame problem around medication is still to be addressed. While ML techniques offer a promising response to the various challenges in medication management, their implementation to help daily care faces many barriers. Data quality is key and must be improved, specifically at the point of capture (standardized data, shared data model, etc.), not only in electronic health records but also for all health-related information (e.g., home electronics). In addition, to fully exploit the potential of ML techniques in medication management, specific challenges need to be addressed to ensure that the tools based on these techniques are effective and can be deployed in daily care. This chapter will present key challenges that must be faced in the development and implementation of ML algorithms for medication management, specifically to estimate exposition to medication, as well as positive and negative outcomes associated with such exposition. Finding ways to describe and include the variability of exposure, and the uncertainty of reactions as part of the development of algorithms will be crucial to make sure the potential can unravel both at the individual and population level.

## 1 The Potential of Machine Learning Techniques for Medication Management

Artificial intelligence (AI) in general, and machine learning (ML) techniques in particular, hold the promise of enormous benefits to medication management, both in the hospital or in the community setting, from clinical decision support (CDS)

A. Motulsky (✉) · J.-N. Nikiema · D. Bosson-Rieutort
Department of Management, Evaluation and Health Policy, School of Public Health of the
Université de Montréal, Montreal, Canada
e-mail: aude.motulsky@umontreal.ca

© Springer Nature Switzerland AG 2021
M. Househ et al. (eds.), *Multiple Perspectives on Artificial Intelligence in Healthcare*,
Lecture Notes in Bioengineering, https://doi.org/10.1007/978-3-030-67303-1_8

to drugs safety and toxicity evaluation (Flynn 2019). Indeed, CDS alerting tools are actually mainly rules-based, and the predefined rules do not take into account the variety of factors (and thus information) involved in the reaction to medications (Challen et al. 2019). This situation leads to the non-consideration of medication errors and adverse reactions by the alerting tools limiting their efficiency in preventing problems.

By their capacity to summarize large amounts of data, ML techniques can be useful to support the medication management process such as validation of prescriptions, by flagging deviant or outlier prescriptions that require attention because they might have an error (Flynn et al. 2019; Schiff et al. 2017). Moreover, ML techniques can be used to generate tools that may learn optimal personalized treatment from real-life data to support continuous medication administration (Nemati et al. 2016; Weng et al. 2017). Then, this potential can help in understanding what matters about the effectiveness and safety of drugs, to support the most important decisions related to medications: Should I take (or prescribe, or authorize?) this medication? (Motulsky 2019; Hernandez and Zhang 2017). And if yes, how?

This is at the convergence of two fields that have been navigating in distinct and parallel universes in the past decades: pharmacoepidemiology and pharmacovigilance. On one side, observational pharmacoepidemiology research has been investigating medication-related outcomes (including effectiveness, cost effectiveness, and adverse events) using various routine data sources such as electronic health records and administrative claims. On the other side, pharmacovigilance, defined as the 'science and activities relating to the detection, assessment, understanding and prevention of adverse effects or any other drug-related problem' (WHO), is required as a pharmacosurveillance activity by regulatory agencies (e.g. FDA, Health Canada). Pharmaceutical companies need to report all adverse events associated with the utilization of their products. These mechanisms are widely based on voluntary reporting by health care organizations, providers and patients who need to declare any adverse reaction associated with a medication. The digital transformation of society in general, and health care in particular, through the explosion of real-life electronic data from various sources (e.g. social media and clinical care), has blurred this frontier between research and post-marketing surveillance (Wei et al. 2019; Wong et al. 2018).

However, while ML techniques offer a promising response to the various challenges in medication management, their implementation to help daily care faces many barriers. Indeed, despite a very wide range of applied methods, in combination or comparison, from naïve Bayesian models, decision trees, to neural networks (Montani and Striani 2019; Basile et al. 2019), there is actually few CDS alerting tools based on ML algorithms. The most evaluated one is MedAware (Segal et al. 2019). Described as more useful than actual implemented rule-based tools, this system has, for now, one major limitation. It cannot take into account unstructured data, like physicians' notes, to find the appropriate information limiting its learning accuracy (Rozenblum et al. 2020). Indeed, the *learning* will only be as good as the data (Lovis 2019; Sgaier and Dominici 2019). The ability to learn from large data becomes obsolete if the algorithm cannot take into account all the available information. This limitation related to the data structure is reflected in research: the most prolific area in the use of ML techniques for medication safety and toxicity evaluation is around Natural Language Processing techniques to detect diagnostics, treatments and adverse drug events in electronic health record (EHR) narratives (Jagannatha et al. 2019; Young et al. 2019; Uzuner et al. 2020).

Thus, access to quality data requires the improvement of health information technology (HIT). Advancing the HIT infrastructure to improve the development and implementation of reliable ML algorithms is not specific to medication management. Data quality must be improved, and the most appropriate way is to do it at the point of capture (standardized data, shared data model, etc.), not only in EHRs but also for all health related information (e.g., home electronics) (Nordo et al. 2019). In addition, to fully exploit the potential of ML techniques in medication management, specific challenges need to be addressed to ensure that the tools based on these techniques are effective and can be deployed in daily care. The objective of this chapter is to present these specific key challenges that must be faced in the development and implementation of ML algorithms for medication management.

## 2 Challenges for the Development of Predictive Analytic Algorithms Related to Medication: Meaningful and Comprehensive Data

Medication-related data are vast and extremely complicated (Motulsky 2019). For data to become 'big', it needs to be aggregated through time and/or space to create massive datasets of persons exposed to medications, and their associated reactions. Consequently, two types of crucial information need to be constructed: (a) data about exposure to medication (who, how, for how long?); and (b) data about reactions to medication, both on the positive and negative sides. The details about these data types and specific challenges will be discussed (Fig. 1).

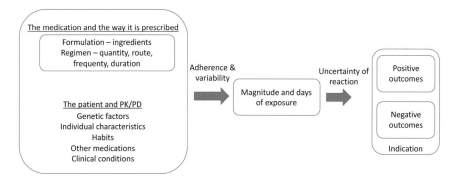

**Fig. 1** Overview of the different type of factors involved in the measure of exposure and reactions to medications

## 2.1  Estimating Medication Exposure

Estimating medication exposure from observational or routine data sources is complicated. Data sources are multiple, and because each has its own limitations and particularities, they are not easy to combine and/or compare. Table 1 presents three types

**Table 1**  Individual-level data required to assess exposure to medication, and their associated data sources and specific challenges

| Type of data sources | Specific challenges |
| --- | --- |
| **Prescription: An order that has been given for a patient to receive a medication** e.g. Citalopram 10 mg per day orally for 6 month | |
| Electronic health or medical records Electronic prescribing systems Electronic prescription repository | The prescription will usually specify the regimen and the duration for this treatment, but not the actual product that is going to be dispensed *Primary adherence*: Medication might be prescribed but the patient will never take it, a phenomenon that is described as primary non adherence. For community dwelling patient, up to 30% of prescriptions written/transmitted are never dispensed to a patient |
| **Dispensation: The product (and quantity) that the patient has received from the pharmacy** e.g. 30 pills of citalopram dispensed on Oct 30 2019 | |
| Pharmacy dispensing records: pharmacy information systems, drug information systems Administrative claims from payers: drug reimbursed to patients | *Secondary adherence*: dispensation does not mean that the medication is taken. The way the patient is actually taking the medication (known as secondary adherence—how and when) is known to be highly variable, especially per therapeutic classes, and associated with patients' characteristics. For inpatients, virtually all prescriptions are dispensed by the pharmacy and administered to the patient. Administration is documented in the electronic patient record through electronic administration record (eMAR) making it easier to map prescription and exposure to the medication. *Generic or other substitutions*: depending on the practices in a given jurisdiction, it might be difficult to infer the product that was given to a patient from a given prescription. For example, the substitution of innovator brand by a generic brand is possible, or the substitution of a solid oral form (e.g. pill) by a liquid oral form (e.g. liquid) is possible, and will not be recorded with the prescription. Multiple formulations from different companies (innovators and generic companies) might not have the same ingredients (other than the therapeutic ingredient), and might be associated with various reactions (e.g. gluten, lactose, etc.) *Contamination*: Examples of contamination of medications by toxic agents through the industrial fabrication processes (e.g. NMDA contamination) is an example of potential contamination of therapeutic products by other chemicals that were not intended to be administered to the patient. |

(continued)

**Table 1** (continued)

| Type of data sources | Specific challenges |
|---|---|
| **Regimen: the dose, route and frequency of the medication to be taken**<br>e.g. Take 10 mg orally every 6 h | |
| *Both prescription or dispensation data sources might include information about the regimen depending on local particularities* | *Computable form*<br>The regimen is used to estimate the daily dose. The regimen is not always documented in a standard and structured format—might be free text only. Moreover, the regimen might be variable, over time, and this makes it difficult to estimate an appropriate daily dose from a given regimen (e.g. 10–20 mg every 4–6 h as needed for 6 months). Days with or without the exposure to the medication are virtually impossible to capture from dispensation data<br>*Pharmacokinetics/pharmacodynamics*<br>The way the molecule is absorbed, distributed in the human body, eliminated through various metabolite forms (that might be involved in adverse reactions), and effective through its pharmacological target, are highly variable depending on the characteristics of the individual patient, such as:<br>• genetic factors: enzymes (cytochromes CYP450, glycoprotein P, etc.) involved in the metabolism (absorption, distribution, elimination) of the drugs; and its pharmacological effect<br>• non genetic factors: age, sex, body weight, size, etc<br>• habits: smoking, diet, physical activity, etc<br>• other medications taken (interactions)<br>• clinical condition(s)<br>Cumulative exposure over time is susceptible to give different exposure profiles and reactions. |

of data that are used to estimate exposure to medications, and specific challenges: prescription, dispensation, and regimen.

The first type of data is about **prescription** that are widely used to estimate exposure to medication. Data sources for prescription includes electronic health records or electronic prescribing systems or repositories, either from an organization, or from an entire nation. However, it is well known that up to 30% of prescriptions are never dispensed for a patient, a phenomenon that is known as primary non adherence (Tamblyn et al. 2014). It is thus very risky to use prescription as a proxy of exposure without taking into account the fact that the patient might never even receive the medication.

The second type of data is about **dispensation**, i.e. what was given to the patient. Dispensation data are closer to the patient, and include information from pharmacy management systems, or data on claims from payers. Here, two types of challenges are important to note. First, secondary non adherence, defined as a divergence from the way the medication is prescribed and the way it is taken by the patient, is very frequent, especially for chronic medications that are supposed to be taken regularly (Bosworth et al. 2011). Dispensation data should not be considered a source of truth for patient exposure to a given medication, and should take into account the uncertainty of exposure. Second, information about the formulation of the product dispensed is required, because different type of substitutions might occur at the pharmacy, depending on the regulation and practices in a given jurisdiction. For example, pharmacists might be allowed to replace an innovator brand by a generic brand for a given molecule, or to replace oral pills for a given molecule by its liquid form. These substitutions are important for two reasons: (1) non therapeutic ingredients might differ from one company to another, leading to variations in many parameters related to drug reactions (e.g. allergic reaction to an excipient used in the preparation of the product) (Page and Etherton-Beer 2018); (2) contamination of specific brands or batch of a given brand by toxic chemicals, such as NMDA, have been detected in the past year (Teasdale 2020). To detect these expositions, details about the batch that has been dispensed to a given patient is required, information that is not always available even in dispensing data currently available.

The third type of information that is required to estimate exposure appropriately is the **regimen** associated with the medication, including the dose (quantity per administration), the route (how the medication will be taken) and the frequency (how many times per day, or per cycle). This information is needed in a standard and structured form to be computable, or different techniques could be used to calculate a daily dose based on free text instructions. However, the regimen might be variable over time, for example when morphine can be taken: 5–10 mg every 4–6 h for 10 days. Or a medication might be prescribed as needed for a few months, and it becomes virtually impossible to define days with and without exposure to medication with precision. Developing techniques to capture this uncertainty is required, to include both adherence and variability of the regimen.

However, the magnitude of the exposure to a specific molecule for a given individual depends on medication and its regimen, but also on the characteristics of this person that are going to influence the way the medication is absorbed, distributed, eliminated (pharmacokinetic profile) and is effective (pharmacodynamic profile). Recently, many pharmacogenomic tests have become popular, especially in mental health and oncology, precisely to identify which individuals are more at risk of either not reacting or overreacting to a specific drug. This is related to the genetic profiles of specific enzymes involved in the metabolism of drugs (e.g. CYP450) or their pharmacological (or clinical) action (e.g. HLA-B 1502 involved in the Steven Johnson life threatening reaction to carbamazepine) (Krebs and Milani 2019). For example, selective serotonin reuptake inhibitors are either primarily metabolized by CYP2C19 (e.g. citalopram, escitalopram) or CYP2D6 (e.g. paroxetine and fluoxetine), which was demonstrated to lead to different types of adverse events (Eugene 2019). Pharmacogenomics is promising a revolution in the way medications are prescribed if your personal profile can be known and your treatment adjusted accordingly (Klein et al. 2017). While individual factors, such as sex, age, weight, or even sociodemographic characteristics, such as income, are more typically collected and used, they are not enough to characterize drug exposure and reaction appropriately. Including genetic factors in the development of ML-based algorithms is important because they can explain a large proportion of differences in terms of reactions to a specific medication, which could be attributed to something else if not considered. The development of an indicator of pharmacogenetic variability of each drug could be part of the solution, to include this uncertainty in the equation.

## 2.2 Estimating Positive and Negative Outcomes in a Computable and Coherent Way

After characterizing exposure to medication, the next step is to characterize the associated reaction to the exposure. These reactions are complicated to define and measure, and this is particularly important for machine-learning based techniques because computers will never know what really matters: how a human being may feel as a result of a given computable observation. A challenge defined by Challen and coll. as the issue of *insensitivity to impact* (Challen et al. 2019). It is thus particularly important to define these outcomes of interest around medication, both on the positive (effectiveness) and the negative (safety) sides.

On the positive side, effectiveness is usually defined as the *degree to which a molecule produces its intended impact under normal or usual circumstances* as opposed to efficacy, which is under ideal (or controlled) conditions. Effectiveness is thus directly linked to intention. To assess whether the medication has helped a patient in a given situation, it is important to know the intention: why was the medication prescribed in the first place? This is what is called the 'indication' or the 'reason for use' of a medication. One could think that this would be easy, because medications are approved for specific indications (e.g. antidepressant should be used for depression, antidiabetic agents should be used for diabetes). However, this is far from being the case, because even if a molecule is approved for a given indication, it could be used for many others—a phenomenon that is called 'off label' usage (to refer to the label that comes with an officially approved medication by regulatory agencies) (Largent 2009). For example, Wong and colleagues (Wong et al. 2016) have demonstrated that 45% of antidepressant medications were prescribed for another indication than depression by general practitioners, and 29% for an indication that was never approved (off-label). The indication would then need to be recorded for each prescription, to group patients based on their intended outcomes. However, indications are rarely documented with prescriptions, making it more complicated to infer if the medication has been effective over time if you do not know what the starting point was (Schiff et al. 2016). Efforts are being pushed forward to document indication in a standard way during the prescribing process (Salmasian et al. 2015), but this practice is not yet associated with most computerized provider order entry systems that are implemented in health care organizations.

Furthermore, most medications are not associated with a systematic, standard and objective measure of positive impact. For example, it is easy to measure blood pressure associated with antihypertensive agents, or triglyceride results associated with lipid-lowering agents. But this is not the case for many agents used in mental health, such as antidepressant agents, that are used for dozens of indications (Wong et al. 2017), antipsychotic agents (e.g. aripiprazole), hypnotic agents (e.g. zaleplon), antinausea agents (e.g. doxylamine-pyridoxine) or antipain agents (e.g. acetaminophen). Nausea, pain or insomnia are only examples of symptoms that are far from being easy to capture in a standard and electronic format. Moreover, many symptoms could be both on the positive side (a symptom that the medication is trying to relieve) and the negative side (a side effect associated with having taken the medication). Making sense of this ocean of data around patients taking (or not taking) medications is one of the biggest challenges of machine learning techniques at the population level. The chronological sequence of the symptom, the exposure to the medication, and the evolution of the symptom over time is key. One could argue that these symptoms are mild, and not life-threatening or critical conditions. But they are part of the equation of how a patient feels when taking a medication, and should not be ruled out when considering the true risk–benefit ratio of a given molecule over time. Not being able to sleep or to drive my car because I am too drowsy might be very important to me. Finding relevant biomarkers or neuroimaging proxies that are associated with specific symptoms is a promising avenue to address this challenge.

On the negative side, adverse events are defined by the WHO as '*a medical occurrence temporally associated with the use of a medicinal product, but not necessarily causally related*' (WHO 2020). They include *side effects*, which are unintended but usually known to be associated with the medication; *adverse reactions*, which are usually unexpected. They may also include errors (accident and incident) that are associated with medication usage. These reactions are rarely documented as part of routine care, unless a dramatic event occurs, or a specific procedure is in place to ensure their systematic documentation. They are usually documented in separated registries managed at a national level, with low integration with clinical data. Regulatory agencies usual maintain registries of reactions that are reported by companies, providers and patients, such as the FDA Adverse Event Reporting System (FAERS). However, these registries are based on voluntary reporting, even if mandatory in some jurisdictions. In other words, very few proactive mechanisms are in place to systematically evaluate if a patient actually feels better when taking a medication in real-life. Recently, real-life data sources (e.g. social media Sarker et al. 2015; Lardon et al. 2015) electronic health records (de Hoon et al. 2017; Li et al. 2018; Wei et al. 2019; Jagannatha et al. 2019) have been used to identify signals of safety events that are rarely documented in a structured and standard way. Issues of confidentiality and privacy then arise.

When defining and selecting outcomes of interest to develop ML-based algorithm, all of these dimensions would ideally need to be included to define the exposure to the medication, and both sides of the reaction to the medication (positive and negative). In the development of algorithms based on ML techniques, one issue is related to the vast number of variables and observations. One strategy to facilitate the creation of algorithms from such large datasets is to reduce dimensionality, i.e. the number of different variables that need to be managed by the algorithm by focusing on the most important variables. This is where it becomes risky in selecting some variables, excluding others, and merging others. For example, Hernandez and colleagues decided to aggregate molecules by therapeutic class instead of keeping the individual molecule separate while investigating the relationship between exposure to antidementia medications and the risk of cardiovascular events (Hernandez 2016). This could lead to inadequate learning because individual molecules in the same therapeutic class could have different safety profiles (Tamblyn et al. 2016). In an algorithm trained to suggest the best medication for treating severe depression, data used to train the algorithm only included treatment response as the positive outcome (symptom resolution), without considering side effects (Benrimoh et al. 2018). Finding the right balance will be key, but crucial information about the formulation, the regimen, the patient and the reactions needs to be considered.

## 3   Conclusion

The potential of machine-learning techniques to support the decision making of patients, clinicians, managers and/or policy-makers is massive. However, the learning will only be as good as the data, and the frame problem around medication is still to be addressed (Challen et al. 2019). Computerized data will always be finite, and will always be covering one portion of the underlying reality and population (Rajkomar et al. 2019). Moreover, humans are highly involved in the creation of any dataset used to train an algorithm, especially in the selection of inputs. Around medication, it is important to make sure that key dimensions are considered to support the development of *responsible* tools, including detailed description of the medication and the patient. Finding ways to describe and include the variability of exposure, and the uncertainty of reactions as part of the development of algorithms will be crucial to make sure the potential can unravel both at the individual and population level.

## References

Basile AO, Yahi A, Tatonetti NP (2019) Artificial intelligence for drug toxicity and safety. Trends Pharmacol Sci 40:624–635

Benrimoh D, Fratila R, Israel S et al (2018) Aifred health, a deep learning powered clinical decision support system for mental health. In: Escalera S, Weimer M (eds) The NIPS '17 competition: building intelligent systems. Springer International Publishing, pp 251–287

Bosworth HB, Granger BB, Mendys P et al (2011) Medication adherence: a call for action. Am Heart J 162:412–424

Challen R, Denny J, Pitt M et al (2019) Artificial intelligence, bias and clinical safety. BMJ Qual Saf 28(3):231–237

de Hoon SEM, Hek K, van Dijk L, Verheij RA (2017) Adverse events recording in electronic health record systems in primary care. BMC Med Inform Decis Mak 17:163

Eugene AR (2019) Optimizing drug selection in psychopharmacology based on 40 significant CYP2C19- and CYP2D6-biased adverse drug reactions of selective serotonin reuptake inhibitors. PeerJ 7:e7860

Flynn A (2019) Using artificial intelligence in health-system pharmacy practice: finding new patterns that matter. Am J Health Syst Pharm 76:622–627

Hernandez I (2016) Risk factors for cardiovascular events of antidementia drugs in Alzheimer's disease patients. J Clin Gerontol Geriatr 7:77–82

Hernandez I, Zhang Y (2017) Using predictive analytics and big data to optimize pharmaceutical outcomes. Am J Health Syst Pharm 74:1494–1500

Jagannatha A, Liu F, Liu W, Yu H (2019) Overview of the first natural language processing challenge for extracting medication, indication, and adverse drug events from electronic health record notes (MADE 1.0). Drug Saf 42:99–111

Klein ME, Parvez MM, Shin J-G (2017) Clinical Implementation of pharmacogenomics for personalized precision medicine: barriers and solutions. J Pharm Sci 106:2368–2379

Krebs K, Milani L (2019) Translating pharmacogenomics into clinical decisions: do not let the perfect be the enemy of the good. Hum Genom 13:39

Lardon J, Abdellaoui R, Bellet F et al (2015) Adverse drug reaction identification and extraction in social media: a scoping review. J Med Internet Res 17:e171

Largent EA (2009) Going off-label without venturing off-course: evidence and ethical off-label prescribing. Arch Intern Med 169:1745

Li F, Liu W, Yu H (2018) Extraction of information related to adverse drug events from electronic health record notes: design of an end-to-end model based on deep learning. JMIR Med Inform 6:e12159

Lovis C (2019) Unlocking the power of artificial intelligence and big data in medicine. J Med Internet Res 21:e16607

Montani S, Striani M (2019) Artificial intelligence in clinical decision support: a focused literature survey. Yearb Med Inform 28:120–127

Motulsky A (2019) Big data challenges from a pharmacy perspective. In: Househ M, Kushniruk AW, Borycki EM (eds) Big data, big challenges: a healthcare perspective: background, issues, solutions and research directions. Springer International Publishing

Nemati S, Ghassemi MM, Clifford GD (2016) Optimal medication dosing from suboptimal clinical examples: a deep reinforcement learning approach. In: 2016 38th annual international conference of the IEEE engineering in medicine and biology society (EMBC), pp 2978–2981

Nordo AH, Levaux HP, Becnel LB et al (2019) Use of EHRs data for clinical research: historical progress and current applications. Learn Health Syst 3:e10076

Page A, Etherton-Beer C (2018) Choosing a medication brand: excipients, food intolerance and prescribing in older people. Maturitas 107:103–109

Rajkomar A, Dean J, Kohane I (2019) Machine learning in medicine. N Engl J Med 380:1347–1358

Rozenblum R, Rodriguez-Monguio R, Volk LA et al (2020) Using a machine learning system to identify and prevent medication prescribing errors: a clinical and cost analysis evaluation. Jt Comm J Qual Patient Saf 46:3–10

Salmasian H, Tran TH, Chase HS, Friedman C (2015) Medication-indication knowledge bases: a systematic review and critical appraisal. J Am Med Inform Assoc 22:1261–1270

Sarker A, Ginn R, Nikfarjam A et al (2015) Utilizing social media data for pharmacovigilance: a review. J Biomed Inform 54:202–212

Schiff GD, Seoane-Vazquez E, Wright A (2016) Incorporating indications into medication ordering-time to enter the age of reason. N Engl J Med 375:306–309

Schiff GD, Volk LA, Volodarskaya M et al (2017) Screening for medication errors using an outlier detection system. J Am Med Inform Assoc JAMIA 24:281–287

Segal G, Segev A, Brom A et al (2019) Reducing drug prescription errors and adverse drug events by application of a probabilistic, machine-learning based clinical decision support system in an inpatient setting. J Am Med Inform Assoc 26:1560–1565

Sgaier S, Dominici F (2019) Using AI to understand what causes diseases. Harv Bus Rev. https://hbr.org/2019/11/using-ai-to-understand-what-causes-diseases. Accessed 18 May 2020

Tamblyn R, Eguale T, Huang A et al (2014) The incidence and determinants of primary nonadherence with prescribed medication in primary care: a cohort study. Ann Intern Med 160:441–450

Tamblyn R, Girard N, Dixon WG et al (2016) Pharmacosurveillance without borders: electronic health records in different countries can be used to address important methodological issues in estimating the risk of adverse events. J Clin Epidemiol 77:101–111

Teasdale A (2020) Regulatory highlights. Org Process Res Dev 24:12–16

Uzuner Ö, Stubbs A, Lenert L (2020) Advancing the state of the art in automatic extraction of adverse drug events from narratives. J Am Med Inform Assoc 27:1–2

Wei Q, Ji Z, Li Z et al (2019) A study of deep learning approaches for medication and adverse drug event extraction from clinical text. J Am Med Inform Assoc JAMIA

Weng W-H, Gao M, He Z et al (2017) Representation and reinforcement learning for personalized glycemic control in septic patients. ArXiv171200654 Cs

WHO quality & safety training course. https://www.who.int/medicines/areas/quality_safety/safety_efficacy/trainingcourses/definitions.pdf. Accessed 18 May 2020

Wong A, Plasek JM, Montecalvo SP, Zhou L (2018) Natural language processing and its implications for the future of medication safety: a narrative review of recent advances and challenges. Pharmacotherapy 38:822–841

Wong J, Motulsky A, Abrahamowicz M et al (2017) Off-label indications for antidepressants in primary care: descriptive study of prescriptions from an indication based electronic prescribing system. BMJ 356:j603

Wong J, Motulsky A, Eguale T et al (2016) Treatment indications for antidepressants prescribed in primary care in Quebec, Canada, 2006–2015. JAMA 315:2230–2232

Young IJB, Luz S, Lone N (2019) A systematic review of natural language processing for classification tasks in the field of incident reporting and adverse event analysis. Int J Med Inf 132:103971

# Reflections on the Clinical Acceptance of Artificial Intelligence

Jens Schneider and Marco Agus

**Abstract** In this chapter, we reflect on the use of Artificial Intelligence (AI) and its acceptance in clinical environments. We develop a general view of hindrances for clinical acceptance in the form of a pipeline model combining AI and clinical practise. We then link each challenge to the relevant stage in the pipeline and discuss the necessary requirements in order to overcome each challenge. We complement this discussion with an overview of opportunities for AI, which we currently see at the periphery of clinical workflows.

## 1 Introduction

To say that Artificial Intelligence (AI) has matured enough over the last decades to be of practical significance would be a clear understatement. As of writing in May 2020, AI is generally regarded as disruptive technology, creating its own job profiles (e.g., Data Scientist), impacting a wide range of industries (e.g., the automotive industry in the form of autonomous vehicles), and spawning new academic programs to cope with the ever increasing demand for skilled man power in the field. Although the Business Insider magazine in 2017 (Business Insider, 2017) listed Healthcare as one out of nine industries that are being transformed by AI around the world, we continue to see what is best described as reluctance in the healthcare sector to fully embrace AI to the extent that other industries already have. But why is that so? Certainly, clinical environments lend themselves to a degree of conservatism, and, one might add, for the better: Many new techniques are not necessarily battle-proven to the standards of clinical rigor. But that alone can hardly explain why, in our opinion, the healthcare sector is slow to adopt to AI-powered technology. To some extent, we agree with the findings of a recent survey on AI-based technology and its use

J. Schneider (✉) · M. Agus
College of Science and Engineering, Hamad Bin Khalifa University, Doha, Qatar
e-mail: jeschneider@hbku.edu.qa

M. Agus
e-mail: magus@hbku.edu.qa

© Springer Nature Switzerland AG 2021                                               103
M. Househ et al. (eds.), *Multiple Perspectives on Artificial Intelligence in Healthcare*,
Lecture Notes in Bioengineering, https://doi.org/10.1007/978-3-030-67303-1_9

to fight COVID-19 (Bullock et al. 2020) that many AI technologies are not yet mature for clinical deployment. However, we believe that this is not a fundamental flaw of the technology itself, but rather the relative lack of well-conducted clinical studies (Wynants et al. 2020). In this chapter, we will therefore analyze reasons for this perceived technological immaturity and factors that hinder clinical acceptance of AI. We will further discuss how these challenges can be overcome, and discuss which types of applications and technologies are more likely to gain acceptance more quickly than others.

## 1.1  AI Nomenclature

This chapter is written from a data science perspective, but targeted at a much broader audience. In an attempt to make this chapter more self-contained, we have therefore taken the liberty to briefly discuss AI nomenclature in this section.

AI can solve different problems, such as *classification* (e.g., given chest x-ray images, does a patient have pneumonia and if so, is it caused by virus or bacteria), various *localization* tasks (e.g., segmentation of structures), processing and interpreting natural languages, etc. The general mechanism is that there is an *architecture* (a term, loosely speaking, relating to the combination of mathematical building blocks, not unlike a popular Danish plastic toy for children) which is home to a plethora of unknown variables. *Training* is then the process to iteratively update these variables by feeding a subset of often annotated data (*training data*) into a robust, numerical optimizer. At the beginning of the training process, variables are initialized with random numbers. The answer to any given query (such as: does this x-ray indicate pneumonia?) will therefore be quite erratic. The deviation between the answer of this mathematical prediction machinery and the known answer or *label* is called the *loss*. Methods using such labels are generally called *supervised* learning—*unsupervised* methods that do not use labelled data are not discussed in this chapter. However, AI is not concerned with memorizing the training data, it is concerned with predicting some aspect of future data samples (class, segments, . . .) it has not encountered before. Therefore, an independent, second data set, the *validation data* is used to ensure the AI can make predictions for unknown data samples. The underlying assumption is that of *statistical generalization*—if the training set is large enough, the insights gained from minimizing the loss generalize to make accurate statements about unknown data from the validation set. The combination of architecture and the numbers learned are called the *model*. The model is the very heart of any AI method, and training good models requires large amounts of data and computational power.

## 2  AI in Clinical Environments

The aforementioned Business Insider article (Business Insider 2017) highlights a UK-based company called Babylon Health that developed a chat-bot based on AI technology such as Natural Language Processing (NLP) that is used by the UK's

National Health Service (NHS) as a contact front-end for patients. Along a similar venue, more specialized chat bots targeting mental health patients in the Arab world have been proposed (Househ et al. 2019a, b), particularly addressing that language barriers may exacerbate the sensitive issue at hand. Albeit not exactly set in a clinical environment, we will analyze in the following why this particular technology seems to have gained acceptance whereas others do not have (yet).

Another application where AI is likely to be integrated into clinical workflows is skin lesion diagnosis using commodity hardware. Driven by the image data made publicly available through the International Skin Imaging Collaboration (ISIC) (ISIC, 2018), the international AI community has picked up the challenge and delivered solutions that achieve accuracy scores above 0.866 (best balanced multiclass accuracy in the ISIC 2018 competition, e.g., Takiddin (2020))—high enough to be of clinical value. In a nutshell, any person with a handheld device such as a smartphone or tablet equipped with a special yet inexpensive clip-on zoom lens can self-diagnose moles and be referred to a MD if necessary. We would like to make two observations regarding this application that we deem important. Firstly, we see the technology developed in this context not so much being used by seasoned dermatologists, but rather by general physicians. The reason is that this technology, for the first time, offers them a way to obtain a second opinion inexpensively, and quickly. It may, therefore, well enter the routine of general physicians to scan their patients, and, if need be, refer them to specialists. Secondly, the innovation behind this technology was driven by rather minuscule incentives (a $4000 cash price for the best entry every year), very similar in style to the now famous DARPA Grand Challenge of 2005 (Buehler et al., 2007), in which a moderate cash prize (in comparison of the US army's monetary efforts up to this point) incentivized the academic, engineering, and technology crowd. It is not only our firm belief that these DARPA challenges had a significant role in kick-starting what has now become the driver-less car industry.

On the other hand, the first author of this chapter briefly worked as an intern in a German university spin-off company developing a computer-based pre-operative planning system for full knee and hip replacements, more than one and a half decades ago. At that time, we were developing an expert system that would recommend position and orientation of implants based on CT scans and a simulation of the ligaments (for the knee replacement). Although similar systems eventually found use at university-affiliated hospitals, certification and registration as a medical device is usually a long and tedious process under most legislations.

We believe that the difference is, mainly, where innovation happens. In both immediate success stories (chatbot and skin lesion diagnosis), innovation happens at "the edge" of the clinical environment, a space that is agile and can pivot quickly. In contrast, the chances for latest technology ("latest" from a research perspective) to be used in "life and death" scenarios is rather scant. The skin lesion system recommends either to see or not to see a physician, and, as long as false negatives can be minimized below the probability of patients not undergoing regular cancer screenings, creates tangible value in a clinical setting. The chatbot developed by Babylon Health essentially streamlines and augments hospital receptions, which may boost productivity while not critically affecting patient treatment. In contrast, full knee or hip prosthetic replacement comprises surgery, and ill-advised prosthetic placement has the potential to affect patients' lifestyle for years to come, including frequent follow-up surgeries. It is, therefore, understandable that exhaustive documentation and studies are normally required for clinical certification and registration of such technology.

The fundamental question, however, is: Do these observations generalize? What are the lessons learned from such anecdotal evidence and how can we further formalize the challenges and opportunities faced in the clinical acceptance of AI-based technology? To understand the problem better, let us sketch how we, from the data science perspective, see the flow from medical data (and all AI is oh so very data hungry) to clinical acceptance, linked to factors potentially hindering this very flow.

## 3 Challenges and Opportunities

Figure 1 summarizes our attempt at a general view of the hindrances affecting clinically approved AI-based technology. In the remainder of this section, will follow the pipeline from data to full clinical acceptance in this figure, we will discuss the challenges associated with each stage and necessary steps to overcome the hindrances.

### 3.1 Data Repositories

As the scenario of skin lesion diagnosis helped motivate, we believe that the first step is to create an inter-institutional data repository. Data is the source of all AI, and the data of one hospital rarely suffices. This, in turn raises questions of data sovereignty and privacy, requiring data to be anonymized in the very least. More subtly, many researchers in the biomedical field grow rather fond of their data, since it represents a substantial investment of time and money on their behalf. Data sovereignty issues may thus potentially be exacerbated by a certain degree of academic mistrust within the community. Another issue obstructing the creation of such repositories are a plethora of incompatible, proprietary, or poorly documented data formats. In the context of the COVID-19 pandemic, one survey explicitly called for the public release of existing case studies (Wynants et al. 2020), finding that this is far from the current practise. We second this and note that in the shadow of the COVID-19 pandemic, we are approaching 5 million cases with over 300,000 deaths as of writing (World Health Organization (WHO) 2020), yet, according to our own research, very few studies seem to have access to large data (e.g., only 1 out of the 15 studies included in a recent survey (Wynants et al. 2020) contained more than 1000 data samples). Furthermore, big companies are collecting their customers' data and may not be willing to share such data on the grounds that this data is key to their own AI endeavours. Regarding clinical or governmental data, academic collaborations can help democratize such

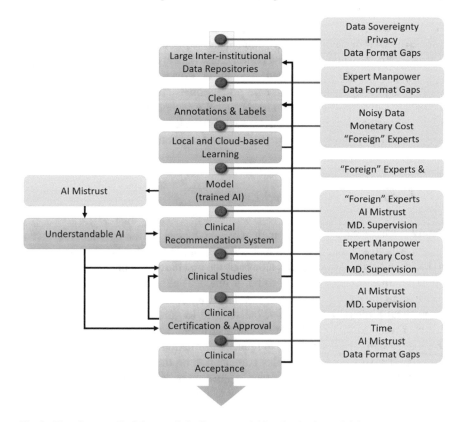

**Fig. 1** Flow from medical data to clinically accepted AI technologies and risks

data and government incentives, Digital or Open Government approaches (OECD 2020) likewise seem adequate mechanism to ensure that the research community has access to large, unbiased, balanced, and diverse data sets. Regarding commercial data, however, the data often represents the commercial edge of tech companies, and the only remedy seems to be careful legislative interventions in which the greater good has to be constantly evaluated against the companies' rights to maintain independent business operations.

## 3.2 Clean Annotation and Labels

Once a repository is created and can be shared with AI researchers, the tedious process of cleaning as well as annotating and labelling the data sets in to provide AIs with a concrete goal for their training. While data scientists may aid in cleaning the data, annotations and labels have to be provided by medical experts. This requires substantial manpower on both the AI and the clinical side. In this and later stages, we assume the view of the clinical environment and view ourselves, the data scientists as "foreign" experts. This shift of view is an exercise mostly motivated by the fact that we commonly see a significant language disconnect or even an outright language barrier between data sciences and health care professionals. This hinders communication and coordination between the two fields. Despite new programs of study targeted at bridging this gap, the authors are not sure if this issue can be successfully overcome in the future, as both fields, and in particular AI, are continuously developing.

## 3.3  Local and Cloud-Based Learning

Finally, we have arrived at the point where a model can be trained. Moderate incentives provided, a clinical problem or challenge could now be outsourced to an army of data scientists and researchers. However, the first hurdle encountered in this stage is that the data is still too noisy to be of practical use. Part of it may actually be attributed to the gap between the medical environment and "foreign" experts. Both the medical profession and data scientists tend to groom their data meticulously. However, the methods could not be more different. Data science models data in clean, quantitative terms, striving to reduce information theoretical redundancy and favoring such structure that enables computation on the data. In contrast, medical data is optimized for human understanding. In a sense, it is richer, more diverse, and, regrettably, tends to be more prone to noise. The reason is that apart from quantitative data, medical professionals also record qualitative data, such as: How does the patient's health improve? What is the pain level? Is the progress better or worse than cases previously encountered by the physician? All these data points are hard to put in numbers, and, physicians consequently prefer to describe their qualitative findings in natural language (with high redundancy), making notes in one of many information systems (data format gap). Consequently, this learning stage may backtrack into the cleaning and data repository steps. Once the data is sufficiently clean, the last hurdle is the monetary cost involved in training AI, sometimes for months on end and on high-end computing hardware. Since much of today's training happens in the cloud, it is important to note that privacy and data sovereignty issues have to be solved before even approaching this stage.

## 3.4  Model (Trained AI)

In this stage, a trained AI is at the fingertips of medical experts and data scientists. Let us assume for now that it does something useful, with an accuracy that is well above uninformed guess work. But how does it actually do it? For sure, we can assume that if we present the AI with the same case it has seen before, it will do its job and return the answer we provided for it in the form of labels. But that is just mere data retrieval; how can we know that the AI is right for a new case, that it *generalizes*? The nagging sensation that the freshly trained AI might be resorting to black magic altogether, called *AI mistrust*, is a very serious hindrance for all stages that follow and a very valid concern (Pollard et al. 2019). A new research direction called understandable AI spawned recently to analyze how the AI actually generalizes from the cases presented to new ones. Researchers in this field try to disassemble and visualize deep networks in order to understand what exactly it is each layer in a deep network does and if the overall network can be trusted. We believe that this field is crucial for the penultimate clinical acceptance of AI, and we would not be surprised if questions regarding explainability and plausibility of the AI as well as the ethical implications of AI were to become mandatory in the clinical certification and approval process in the near future (Sloane and Silva 2020).

## 3.5 Clinical Recommendation System

Assume you are a data scientist and you have successfully overcome all the hurdles so far. You have trained a model from clinically relevant data and you have built a recommendation system that uses AI. You would, of course, like to advertise it as a panacea that automatically diagnoses a wide range of diseases or makes recommendations so profound that you fully expect it to replace squadrons of medical professionals within the next couple of months. But you are aware of the ethical implications and you suspect you have succumbed to hubris of the advanced kind. Therefore, you humbly state that a physician has to verify the result of your AI and has to decide its use in any clinical treatment. In short, your system advises a physician whereas the physician supervises your system. It therefore becomes a *tool*, with liability implications that we will discuss later in this chapter. This scenario is of value, to varying degrees, depending on the context. If the recommendation system operates at the non-critical edge of the healthcare system, it may end up adding significant value. If it is targeted at the core of the health care system (e.g., operation theaters where time is extremely valuable and experience is everything), it may never be accepted. We believe that the key to understanding this difference are two simple questions: How much time does the supervisor have/is willing to spend in order to get an advise? How much time will the advice potentially save or how much will it improve the patient's and doctor's life? Going back to the example of skin lesion diagnosis: The AI is a recommendation system that sits at the edge of the health care system. It does not cost much time or effort and simply provides a second opinion. The risk of not treating a range of skin cancers in a range of patients will most likely convince many non-dermatologists to use this system. Dermatologists may evaluate the technology based on its accuracy and the amount of time the AI saves for them.

## 3.6   Clinical Studies

The next stage are clinical studies. This stage requires expert manpower, time, money, and supervision through healthcare professionals. In this context, clinical studies should not only assess whether the AI is reliable and accurate, but they should also try to assess the ethical and social implications of using an AI. Are physicians and patients comfortable with taking advice of an AI? Will the AI be in direct contact with patients or only the professionals? What is the improvement in the professionals' workflows? Do they actively supervise the technology or do they grow fatigued and accept the advice uncritically?

## 3.7   Clinical Certification and Approval

This stage essentially takes AI from research to a medical product. Understandably, this step takes time and requires substantial involvement of physicians, lawyers, data scientists, etc. Since systems for clinical use have to be fully documented, again AI mistrust may be a hurdle that can be overcome by demonstrating that the AI is plausible and understandable. It is worth noting though that the time required to achieve approval generally translates into technology out-dating in the process. This is all the more true for AI-based solutions which are fueled by one of the fastest growing research fields at the moment.

## 3.8   Clinical Acceptance

We do not equate the mere fact that an AI has undergone certification and has been approved to clinical acceptance. We define clinical acceptance as:

> A significant portion of major hospitals has heard of a technology and either considers its use or is using that technology.

Again, there are a wide range of reasons why an approved technology would not become accepted. For instance, the manufacturer of a product is unable to integrate the product into a hospital's workflow or IT infrastructure (data format gap), the hospital is not convinced about the benefits of AI-based products (AI mistrust), or the product is simply too new to be widely accepted.

## 3.9   Liability Risks

Even though AI is still far from being largely accepted in core clinical setups, we feel that it is important to mention potential issues related to legal liability in addition to the risks outlined in Fig. 1. We consider this in some ways very similar to the liability issues posed by recent advancements in autonomous driving vehicles (Kingston 2016), or all artificially intelligent computer systems. The main general questions can be summarized as follows:

- Who is liable (AI developer vs. medical practitioner)?
- Whether and when shall criminal or civil code be applied (e.g., for malpractice)?
- Is AI is an instrument, a tool, a service, or more?

The interaction between physicians who tend to see AI as tools and the AI developers boils down to the following conflict: neither party wants to accept liabilities. This is probably one of the reasons clinical approval processes are so involved. We believe that, in order to understand liability better, we have to distinguish between the following scenarios:

- Medical malpractice, in which physicians risk law suits from patients who feel that the physicians were negligent in their treatment.
- Uncritical and uncontrolled reliance on automatic diagnosis and treatment decisions.
- Technical malpractice, in which AI achieves clinical certification despite undocumented, untested, or overlooked erratic behaviour that can lead to wrong decisions.

While it seems that clinicians tend to blame responsibility for wrong decisions on system providers, the same system provides tend to contractually exclude such liabilities. Therein lies a dilemma that will generate many future law controversies (Braun et al. 2020). To this end, the European Commission has very recently faced this delicate issue and published a report that looks at whether the existing liability regimes are sufficient for the purposes of attributing liability in relation to highly complex tools such as AI and emerging technologies (The European Commission 2019, 2020). The report highlights that a person using a technology that has a certain degree of autonomy should not be less accountable for harm caused than if said harm had been caused by a human aide. However, as AI technology will continue to evolve, we believe that the existing legislative framework for tort and product liability will need to be adapted accordingly. In the meantime, all stakeholders will need to assess whether or not they are sufficiently protected against liability risks arising from usage of AI, be it as operators, users, or manufacturers. This could be by way of contractual arrangements (e.g. warranties and indemnities), or by taking out appropriate insurance coverage. From our point of view, we do not feel in the position of expressing an opinion on these delicate issues. However, we wanted to point out that we firmly believe that, when an AI-based decision support system is planned to be used in a clinical environment, a deep discussion is necessary at different levels to define specific responsibilities, starting from design specifications, to product implementation, and usage instructions and limitations.

# 4 Conclusion

Given all these considerations, we believe that the greatest opportunities for AI are currently on the edge of the healthcare system. Here, AI-powered applications can bypass full medical certification since they are not yet mission critical. Challenges of data sovereignty and privacy remain, but AI targeted at this segment may also well pave the way for a wider base of AI acceptance in the patient population. Considering that AI and data science have become much more accessible during the last few years due to major advances in API design, another way to bridge the gap between data science and medical profession would be to further abstract typical algorithmic tasks, like the training and validation process, in a way to enable physicians with no coding experience to build automated deep learning models that might once have been out of reach (Pollard et al. 2019). This may be further assisted by data scientists already on pay roll in large hospitals. Being exposed to the way AIs are designed might also help in reducing AI mistrust.

The largest challenge we see is the need to democratize data. The largest and most valuable source of data in healthcare arguably comes from Electronic Medical/Health Records (EMRs/EHRs). However, clinician satisfaction with EMRs is still very low, with regards to completeness and quality of data entries (Melnick et al. 2020). This is made worse by inter-operability issues between different providers. At the same time, EMRs raise an interesting question: who owns the data in the EMR? Clearly, patients contribute their private data to an EMR, so there is at least partial ownership. However, also the physicians contribute to the EMR in the form of diagnoses, prescriptions, etc. Should, therefore, hospitals also assume partial ownership of the EMR? We believe not, since they were paid for their service and, therefore become consultants to their patients. We cannot rule out that this assessment might be wishful thinking from a data scientist perspective though, since it would imply that patients can voluntarily disclose all the data collected in their EMRs and all their history stored at hospitals into public or third party repositories, such as the now defunct Google Health or likewise defunct Microsoft HealthVault (Morley et al. 2019). Questions such as these, of data ownership, liability distribution, responsibility and permission to use are at the very core of realizing the full potential of AI across health systems. In general, we can expect that the prevalent scenario for data infrastructure development will depend more on the socio-economic context of the health system in question rather than on technology. In the current status, the potential of AI is sufficiently highlighted, but in reality, health systems are faced with a dilemma: to significantly reduce the enthusiasm regarding the potential of AI in everyday clinical practice, or to resolve issues of data ownership, liability and trust, and to invest in the data infrastructure to realize it (Panch et al. 2019). Such considerations will, eventually, tie back to and define AI ethics, a field currently emerging in academia.

# References

Braun M, Hummel P, Beck S, Dabrock P (2020) Primer on an ethics of AI-based decision support systems in the clinic. J Med Ethics. https://doi.org/10.1136/medethics-2019-105860

Buehler M, Iagnemma K, Singh S (2007) The 2005 DARPA Grand Challenge: The Great Robot Race. Springer, 2007 ed. ISBN 978-3540738284

Bullock J, Luccioni A, Pham KH, Lam CSN, Luengo-Oroz M (2020) Mapping the landscape of artificial intelligence applications against COVID-19. arXiv:2003.11336v2. Accessed 18 May 2020

Business Insider (2017) From A to I: how 9 industries are being transformed by UK innovation around the world. https://www.businessinsider.com/sc/artificial-intelligence-companies?IR=T#group-h-YWTfUA1oOU. Accessed 18 March 2020

Househ M, Alam T, Al-Thani D, Schneider J, Siddig MA, Fernandez-Luque L, Qaraqe M, Al-Fuqaha A, Saxena S (2019a) Developing a digital mental health platform for the Arab world: from research to action. Stud Health Technol Inform 262:392–395. https://doi.org/10.3233/SHTI190101

Househ M, Schneider J, Ahmad K, Alam T, Al-Thani D, Siddig MA, Fernandez-Luque L, Qaraqe M, Al-Fuqaha A, Saxena S (2019b) An evolutionary bootstrapping development approach for a mental health conversational agent. Stud Health Technol Inform 262:228–231. https://doi.org/10.3233/SHTI190060

ISIC (2018) International Skin Imaging Collaboration. https://www.isic-archive.com/. Accessed 18 March 2020

Kingston JK (2016) Artificial intelligence and legal liability. In: International Conference on Innovative Techniques and Applications of Artificial Intelligence, pp 269–279. Springer. https://doi.org/10.1007/978-3-319-47175-4_20

Melnick ER, Dyrbye LN, Sinsky CA, Trockel M, West CP, Nedelec L, Tutty MA, Shanafelt T (2020) The association between perceived electronic health record usability and professional burnout among us physicians. Mayo Clinic Proceedings 95(3):476–487. https://doi.org/10.1016/j.mayocp.2019.09.024

Morley J, Taddeo M, Floridi L (2019) Google Health and the NHS: overcoming the trust deficit. Lancet Digital Health 1(8):e389. https://doi.org/10.1016/S2589-7500(19)30193-1

OECD (2020) Open Government. https://www.oecd.org/gov/open-government/. Accessed 18 May 2020

Panch T, Mattie H, Celi LA (2019) The "inconvenient truth" about AI in healthcare. npj Digital Med 2:77. https://doi.org/10.1038/s41746-019-0155-4

Pollard TJ, Chen I, Wiens J, Horng S, Wong D, Ghassemi M, Mattie H, Lindemer E, Panch T (2019) Turning the crank for machine learning: ease, at what expense? The Lancet Digital Health 1(5):e198–e199. https://doi.org/10.1016/S2589-7500(19)30112-8

Sloane EB, Silva RJ (2020) Artificial intelligence in medical devices and clinical decision support systems. In: Clinical Engineering Handbook, pp 556–568. Elsevier. https://doi.org/10.1016/B978-0-12-813467-2.00084-5

Takiddin A (2020) An artificial intelligence tool to detect and classify skin cancer, vol 4. MS thesis, College of Science and Engineering, Hamad Bin Khalifa University, Doha, Qatar

The European Commission (2019) Liability for artificial intelligence and other emerging digital technologies. The European Commission. https://ec.europa.eu/transparency/regexpert/index.cfm?do=groupDetail.groupMeetingDoc&docid=36608. Accessed 18 May 2020

The European Commission (2020) White paper on artificial intelligence—a European approach to excellence and trust. The European Commission. https://ec.europa.eu/info/sites/info/files/commission-white-paper-artificial-intelligence-feb2020_en.pdf. Accessed 18 May 2020

World Health Organization (WHO) (2020) Coronavirus disease (COVID-19) pandemic. https://www.who.int/emergencies/diseases/novel-coronavirus-2019?gclid=EAIaIQobChMIyo6D8re96QIVx6qWCh1vcQGIEAAYASAAEgK3zvD_BwE. Accessed 18 May 2020

Wynants L, Calster BV, Bonten MMJ, Collins GS, Debray TPA, Vos MD, Haller MC, Heinze G, Moons KGM, Riley RD, Schuit E, Smits LJM, Snell KIE, Steyerberg EW, Wallisch C, van Smeden M (2020) Prediction models for diagnosis and prognosis of covid-19 infection: systematic review and critical appraisal. BMJ 369. https://doi.org/10.1136/bmj.m1328

# Artificial Intelligence for Chatbots in Mental Health: Opportunities and Challenges

Kerstin Denecke, Alaa Abd-Alrazaq, and Mowafa Househ

**Abstract** With the help of artificial intelligence, the way humans are able to understand each other and give a response accordingly, is fed into the chatbot systems, i.e. into systems that are supposed to communicate with a user. The bot understands the user's query and triggers an accurate response. In the healthcare domain, such chatbot based systems gain in interest since they promise to increase adherence to electronically delivered treatment and disease management programmes. In this chapter, we provide an overview on chatbot systems in mental health. Artificial intelligence is exploited in such systems for natural language understanding, to create a human-like conversation and to make appropriate recommendations given a specific user utterance and mental state. Potential benefits of chatbots have been shown with respect to psychoeducation and adherence. However, there are also limitations and ethical issues to be considered including the impact on the patient-therapist relationship, the risk of over-reliance or the limited skills and emotional intelligence of chatbots that might limit their applicability.

## 1 Introduction

A chatbot is a system that interacts with users using natural language (written or spoken) or facial expressions and body language (Sansonnet et al. 2006). Other terms that have been used for a chatbot include: machine conversation system, virtual agent, dialogue system, conversational user interface (CUI), and chatterbot. The purpose of a chatbot system is to simulate a human conversation. Chatbots are usually text-driven,

K. Denecke (✉)
Institute for Medical Informatics, Bern University of Applied Sciences, Bern, Switzerland
e-mail: kerstin.denecke@bfh.ch

A. Abd-Alrazaq · M. Househ
Division of Information and Computing Technology, College of Science and Engineering,
Hamad Bin Khalifa University, Qatar Foundation, Doha, Qatar
e-mail: aabdalrazaq@hbku.edu.qa

M. Househ
e-mail: mhouseh@hbku.edu.qa

© Springer Nature Switzerland AG 2021
M. Househ et al. (eds.), *Multiple Perspectives on Artificial Intelligence in Healthcare*,
Lecture Notes in Bioengineering, https://doi.org/10.1007/978-3-030-67303-1_10

with images and unified widgets, which makes it easy to start interacting with a bot. There are two types of chatbots: unintelligent (rule-based) chatbots which generate their dialogue based on some predefined rules or decision trees, and intelligent chatbots which use Artificial Intelligence (AI) to understand the context and intent of a user utterance and respond to it (Hussain et al. 2019). Our focus in this chapter is on intelligent chatbots that use AI.

Chatbots have been used in health-related applications for example to achieve a health behaviour change (Fadhil and Gabrielli 2017) or to support disease self-management. Healthcare chatbots support patients, families of patients or the healthcare team by providing specific knowledge, therapy support (e.g. Wysa provides cognitive behaviour therapy (Inkster et al. 2018)) or help in managing diseases (e.g. eMMA helps in managing medications (Tschanz et al. 2018)). Many chatbot-based applications exist for supporting mentally ill people. As an example, this chapter concentrates on chatbots for this particular use case.

Mental disorders may influence 29% of people in their lifetime (Steel et al. 2014) and may affect 25% of adults and 10% of children in a year (Mental Health Foundation 2015). In addition that mental disorders decrease the quality of people's lives, they are considered one of the most common causes of disability (Whiteford et al. 2015). It has been estimated that mental disorders will produce costs of $16 trillion between 2011 and 2030 due to lost labour and capital output (Jones et al. 2014).

Mental disorders are normally treated by pharmacotherapy or psychotherapy (Cuijpers et al. 2013). However, there is a global shortage of mental health human resources with demand out-stripping service provision. There are nine psychiatrists per 100,000 people available in developed countries (Murray et al. 2012), whereas there is one psychiatrist for every ten million people in developing countries (Oladeji and Gureje 2016). According to the WHO, about 45% of people in developed and 15% of people in developing countries, can reach mental health services (Anthes 2016). Leaving people with mental disorders untreated may increase suicidal attempts and mortality (Hester 2017).

To address this matter of limited resources for treating persons with mental disorders, conversational agents gained in interest in the last years in particular for psychoeducation, behaviour change and self-help (Bendig et al. 2019). In this way, they are used to offer fully automated self-help services. This chapter provides an overview on the characteristics of mental health chatbots and discusses the benefits and challenges of such systems.

## 2  Chatbots for Mental Health

### 2.1  Overview of Chatbots for Mental Health

According to a review conducted by Abd-alrazaq and colleagues (2019), there are 41 different chatbots for mental health reported by 53 studies. About 43% of those chatbots were implemented in the United States of America. They have been developed for different purposes, namely: therapy (e.g. Woebot), training (e.g. LISSA), and screening (e.g. SimSensei), focusing on depression and autism. The majority of chatbots (70%) were implemented as stand-alone software whereas a minority of chatbots was implemented as web-based platforms. Approximately 89% of the identified chatbots are rule-based, i.e. use predefined rules or decision trees to generate chatbot responses. The remaining chatbots utilise AI to generate responses. In 87% of the studies, the dialogues are controlled and led by the chatbots only, whereas the dialogue was controlled by both chatbots and users in 7 studies. The majority of chatbots had embodiment on their screens such as an avatar or virtual human.

As examples for this large landscape of mental health chatbots, we will briefly describe two mental health chatbots (Wysa and SERMO). Wysa is an emotional and intelligent chatbot (Inkster et al. 2018). It integrates a mood tracker and can detect negative moods. Depending on the mood of the client, it suggests a depression test and recommends seeking professional help depending on the outcome of the test. For supporting the relief of anxiety, depression and stress, there are mindfulness meditation exercises integrated in the app. The chatbot was tested in a study with a total of 129 participants, who were divided into two groups (frequent and occasional users) (Inkster et al. 2018). The quantitative results show that frequent users had a higher, average improvement in their mood than the group of occasional users ($P >$ 0.03) (Inkster et al. 2018). Two thirds of the users perceived the app as positive. They confirmed that the conversation with Wysa was helpful and stimulating (Inkster et al. 2018).

SERMO is a mobile application for people with a slight psychological impairment (Denecke et al. 2020). It implements methods from cognitive behaviour therapy (CBT) and supports in regulating emotions and dealing with thoughts and feelings. The application comprises a conversational agent that asks the user on a daily basis on events that occurred, his thoughts and feelings. The ABC theory (situation, thoughts, emotions) by Albert Ellis has been implemented into the chatbot for this purpose. The theory follows the approach that consciously or unconsciously perceived stimuli are evaluated and these evaluations lead to certain feelings and behaviours (Wilken 2015). From the collected information, SERMO determines automatically the basic emotion of a user from natural language input. So far, five emotions can be recognized: fear, anger, grief, sadness, and happiness. Depending on the emotion, an appropriate measurement such as activities or mindfulness exercises is suggested by the system. Additional functions are an emotion diary, a list of pleasant activities, mindfulness exercises and information on emotions and CBT in general. The chatbot has been implemented using the OSCOVA framework (http://oscova.com). For a prototype, 13 dialogs have been developed with OSCOVA. They cover the various interactions triggered by an emotion or mood expressed by the user. It can be considered as a decision tree that is processed depending on the user interaction. Emotions are detected and classified using natural language processing methods and lexicon-based procedures. In this respect, SERMO is a hybrid approach of a chatbot, integrating a rule-based conversation flow with natural language understanding capabilities. SERMO was evaluated regarding user experience with 21 users (mentally impaired patients and psychologists) using the User Experience Questionnaire (UEQ). Findings show that efficiency, perspicuity and attractiveness are considered as good. The scales describing hedonic quality (stimulation and novelty), i.e., fun of use, show neutral evaluations. The involved experts confirmed that the app is well suited for patients with problems in expressing themselves in a face-to-face encounter. They see potentials that a chatbot could well bridge the gap between two therapeutic sessions (instead of calling the therapist, the patient could chat with SERMO). However, they suggested that a therapist should receive an alert when the system determines a certain risk for a patient from the conversations.

## 2.2   Role of AI in Mental Health Chatbots

First approaches to chatbots required the programmer to define a set of possible user inputs and corresponding replies for the chatbot (Weizenbaum 1966). For this purpose, corresponding literature has to be reviewed in order to create a chatbot that utilizes that evidence-based medical knowledge. For encapsulating this knowledge in the "brain" of the chatbot, scripting languages such as Artificial Intelligence Markup Language (http://www.aiml.foundation/) or Rivescript (https://www.rivescript.com/) have been used for this purpose (Rahman et al. 2017). In the last few years, AI has been applied to make a chatbot conversation human-like. More specifically, with the help of AI, the way humans are able to understand each other and give a response accordingly, is fed into the chatbot systems. Frameworks that support development of AI-based chatbots are for example OSCOVA (https://oscova.com), IBM Watson or RASA stack (https://rasa.com).

AI provides two elements to enable chatbots providing an appropriate response to a user statement: machine learning and natural language processing (NLP) (Abdul-Kader and Woods 2015). Machine learning algorithms are used to learn from data, either from training data or from the previous conversation with a bot, to recognize patterns, or monitor the past which helps in generating an appropriate response (Shawar and Atwell 2005). The underlying training data has to be comprehensive to cover a diverse mixture of conversation flows and aspects as well as user statements. In recent years, deep learning became a buzz word and is increasingly used to be included into chatbots where a predefined set of responses is not desirable or workable (Csaky 2019). Deep learning is a type of machine learning that uses layered algorithms called an artificial neural network (Lauzon 2012). It involves techniques to discover representations in the data that allow it to make sense of raw data. Each layer of algorithms, in turn, comprises interconnected artificial neurons. The connections between these neurons are weighted by the prior learning patterns and events. The algorithms find patterns in vast quantities of data and infer how to respond to new data from these patterns.

NLP methods target at analysing the natural language user input. They help a system in understanding and interpreting user input, detects patterns in a user statement, identifies entities, co-occurrences, or determines relations. Tasks include domain classification (about which topic is a user talking?), determining the user intent and slot filling (Jurafsky and Martin 2008). The analysis results are required to create an appropriate response of the chatbot since they aim at determining intents, emotions and other semantics hidden in a user statement.

From the chatbot examples presented before, it can be recognized already what AI is doing in mental health chatbots (Lovejoy 2019). Natural language processing is applied for analysing user utterances, for summarizing the utterances, for identifying significant changes, for sentiment or emotion analysis, or entity recognition (Denecke et al. 2020). Analysed user input can be used with comprehensive machine learning algorithms to predict outcomes or behaviour changes or to timely identify them (e.g. the risk for suicide or self harm determined based on the user interaction). AI in mental health chatbots is required for generating appropriate responses of the chatbots or selecting adequate measurement to be suggested to the user (Gao et al. 2019). Input to the AI algorithms are the results from the conversation analysis, but can be extended by data from other sources such as sensors available in a mobile phone. Sensor data such as data from activity tracker provide additional indicators for recognizing changes in behaviour or for predicting risks (Lovejoy 2019; Chung and Park 2019). By learning from the different data items recommendations can be personalized to a larger extent.

Building AI-based chatbots requires training data which is difficult to generate and it is more difficult to ensure that AI-based chatbots generate adequate responses or even to control their responses. These might be reasons why AI is rarely used in available chatbots for mental health.

## 3   Benefits of Chatbots in Mental Health

This section summarizes benefits of mental health chatbots. Clearly, there are negative aspects or challenges. They will be outlined in Sect. 4. Chatbots are able to alleviate the issue of a global shortage of mental health human resources as they are usually available to millions of users at anytime and anywhere—especially in war zones where many serious mental disorders occur (Luxton 2020). This, in turn, has the potential to improve the availability and quality of mental healthcare at reduced expenses.

In addition, chatbots are suitable for providing mental health treatment for those who find it difficult to disclose their mental issues to a healthcare provider due to stigmatization. According to Lucas and colleagues, veterans disclosed more symptoms of posttraumatic stress disorder to a chatbot than anonymized and non-anonymized versions of a self-administrated questionnaire (Lucas et al. 2017).

Given that chatbots typically use easy-to-use interfaces and interact with users using different input and output modalities, they are appropriate for users with low computer, health, and reading literacy skills. A study showed that a wide range of users, including those who have never used computers before, found chatbots easy to use (Bickmore et al. 2005).

Embodied chatbots can interact with users using verbal and nonverbal behaviours and show empathy, concentration, and close proximity. This, in turn, enables them to establish a therapeutic alliance with patients.

Although usual computerized interventions can be effective in improving mental health, they are characterized by high dropout rates and poor adherence owing to the lack of the quality of human interaction that face-to-face encounters with healthcare providers offer (Nooijer et al. 2005; Grolleman et al. 2006). Chatbots can become a promising alternative to those interventions through their intuitive, human-like, and entertaining interaction with users, thereby, they can improve users' adherence (Grolleman et al. 2006).

Previous studies showed many potential benefits of using chatbots for mental health. Specifically, chatbots are effective in improving several mental health issues. For example, studies showed that there is a statistically significant difference favouring chatbots over reading an eBook on the severity of depression ($P = 0.017$) (Fitzpatrick et al. 2017) and anxiety ($P = 0.02$) (Fulmer et al. 2018). Chatbots have the potential to teach mentally-ill people social skills (e.g. job interviewing skills) and allow them to practice these skills in a non-judgmental environment. For instance, chatbot users showed significantly higher improvement than the waiting-list group on job interview skills ($P < 0.05$) and self-confidence ($P < 0.05$) (Smith et al. 2014). Chatbots have the potential to detect several mental issues. Ujiro and colleagues (Ujiro et al. 2018) developed a chatbot to detect patients with dementia, and they found high performance of the chatbot in detecting dementia (area under the curve (AUC) of 95%).

# 4 Challenges

Even though there are multiple benefits of using AI in mental health chatbots, there are also challenges on different levels to be considered. We distinguish technical challenges, ethical challenges, challenges of practical implementation, and accountability implications.

## 4.1 Technical Limitations of Mental Health Chatbots

Even though AI can realize already good conversations and help in creating chatbots that pass the Turing test, there are still technical limitations. Existing systems are unable to remember what has been said in previous conversations, which might lead to inappropriate responses (Abd-alrazaq et al. 2020a). Knowledge on the user and his/her mental state has to be collected and stored for future interactions with the bot to address this issue. A chatbot reply might be frustrating or inadequate for a user due to a lack of understanding or missing emotional intelligence (Abd-alrazaq et al. 2020a). The skills of existing mental health chatbots are generic, often repetitive and the interaction is often similar to a self-help book (Abd-alrazaq et al. 2020a). Altogether, this might cause annoyance and limits user adherence to such applications.

Existing mental health chatbots are often authored systems, guiding through a predefined conversation flow. When mental health chatbots become self-learning systems through integration with AI, the systems might develop own rules and make own decisions which are out of control of an evidence-based interaction or might even create harm in patients. For example, a Microsoft chatbot started to insult people after some time, which it was not expected to do (Baer 2016). The reason was that the system was tricked by users.

Another important issue for the development of AI-based mental health chatbots is that AI algorithms are normally trained on large data sets. Other approaches that require less training data or use transfer learning are under development, but again, training on data from other domains might introduce knowledge into the system that might risk patient harm. Further, trained models can become biased towards certain population groups when the underlying training data is insufficiently sampled or data is unavailable for some sub-groups. A challenge here is that existing research does not study in depth the technical limitations of the developed mental health chatbots (Abd-alrazaq et al. 2020b; Laranjo et al. 2018). Evaluations basically assess usability and user experience (Abd-alrazaq et al. 2020b; Laranjo et al. 2018).

## 4.2 Ethical Challenges

There are many mental health chatbots available in the app stores; however, many of them are not evidence-based or at least the underlying knowledge is not undermined by relevant research (Kretzschmar et al. 2019). In order to be reliable and efficient, mental health chatbots should rely upon clinical evidence, i.e. clinical approaches have to be integrated that are already in use in clinical practice and have shown effectiveness. Further, there is only limited evidence on the therapeutic effect of mental health chatbots (Miller and Polson 2019; Vaidyam et al. 2019). According to a systematic review, it is difficult to draw definitive conclusions regarding the effect of chatbots on several mental health outcomes due to a high risk of bias in the included studies, low quality of evidence, lack of studies assessing each outcome, small sample size in the included studies, and contradictions in results of some included studies (Abd-alrazaq et al. 2020c). Such limitations may harm users by inappropriate recommendations or unrecognized risks (Luxton 2020).

Given the sensitivity of users' data about their mental well-being, chatbots must keep them private and confidential (Stiefel 2018). Unlike patient-doctor encounters, where patient privacy and confidentiality are protected, chatbots often do not consider these aspects. Most chatbots, especially those are available on social media platforms, do not allow users to chat anonymously (Luxton et al. 2016). Therefore, conversations can be linked to users. Several chatbots explicitly stated in their terms and conditions that they can exploit and share their data for different purposes. However, users often accept such terms and conditions presented in a dense and formal language without careful reading, thereby, they may not be aware that their data will not be kept confidential. This means the data could be sold, traded or marketed by the distributor of a chatbot. The best example of this is the Facebook scandal, when Facebook shared data for millions of users with Cambridge Analytica without their consent. Cyber-attacks might become another issue that will make user's personal health data available for unknown purposes. Altogether, these issues impact on the users' acceptance of chatbots and quantity of sensitive data shared by them.

Safety is another challenge of using chatbots. Currently, most chatbots lack the ability to manage emergency situations, where users' safety is at risk (Kretzschmar et al. 2019). This may be attributed to the inability of chatbots to contextualize users' conversations, to grasp their emotional cues, and to remember their previous conversations. Although some chatbots (e.g. Wysa) offer the option of getting instant support by a mental health professional, such services are usually not free and inaccessible by those who are younger than 18 years. Over-reliance on chatbots is another issue related to safety. In other words, users of chatbots may become overattached to or over-reliant on them due to their ease of access, thereby, this may increase their addictive behaviours and lead them to avoid face-to-face visits with mental health professionals (Kretzschmar et al. 2019; Vaidyam et al. 2019).

AI chatbots always endeavour to pass the Turing test by making users think that they are talking to human rather than a machine. Patients are deceived into believing the chatbot is real by equipping the chatbot with empathy and by responses that create the impression of talking to a human. Also reflecting exactly behaviour of therapists might intensify this impression. However, from a healthcare perspective, this deception may be considered as unethical as users have a right to know with whom they are interacting. In some cultures, interacting with a computer or robot instead of a human may even be deemed insulting. To avoid this ethical dilemma, Kretzschmar and colleagues (Kretzschmar et al. 2019) recommended chatbot developers to inform and keep reminding users that they are interacting with a machine with limited capacity to understand users' needs. Most chatbots are also not able to show real empathy or sympathy, which are very important elements of psychotherapy. Therefore, many people may not be comfortable with using such chatbots in mental healthcare.

Finally, we are missing ethical and regulatory frameworks for mHealth interventions in general and mental health applications in particular; there is potential for misuse of chatbot technology including using the technologies to replace established services, thereby potentially exacerbating existing health inequalities (Fiske et al. 2019). Recent work tries to address these issues: A consensus statement around standards for mental health apps has been developed by a group of patients, physicians, researchers, insurance organisations, technology companies and the US National Institute of Mental Health programme officers (Torous et al. 2019). Their consensus consider standards for: (a) data safety and privacy, (b) effectiveness, (c) user experience/adherence, (d) data integration.

## 4.3 Impact on User and Healthcare Team

Physicians and therapists recognize positive and negative aspects of the use of health chatbots, including the support in managing one's own health and benefits on psychological and behavioural health outcomes (Palanica et al. 2019). Chatbots cannot effectively care for all patient needs, cannot display human emotions. They might be helpful in less complicated tasks such as administrative and organizational tasks or data collection tasks, but as soon as comprehensive knowledge on a patient is needed, they might fail (Palanica et al. 2019). Repetitive administrative tasks could be well realized and have the potential of freeing time for physicians or therapists to provide care to their patients. Consider as an example a chatbot that generates a mood diary from daily interaction with a user. The collected information could be aggregated by AI in a way that the therapist can recognize significant changes in the mood, even associated with activity data that is recorded. This provides an additional information source to the therapist and can improve the recommendations and therapy.

It is still unclear whether the patient-therapeutic relationship gets impacted by the adoption of chatbots into mental healthcare. With a chatbot as a second opinion or a companion who is available all the time—is this an opponent to the real-world therapist? A solution to avoid a critical impact on the relationship might be to integrate it carefully into the care plan (Miller and Polson 2019). This includes also that the chatbot should be able to recognize critical situations and should refer to the physician. Experiences on this are still unavailable in the research literature. As mentioned before, a huge problem in current practice is that too many people don't have access to mental health services. In this context, chatbots could at least provide some help. Long-term use might impact patient's behaviour and strategies in seeking help. People might start preferring emotional support from the machine instead of their friends and families (Miller and Polson 2019). In this way, the chatbot use can lead to a loss of personal contacts and loss of capabilities of dealing with conflicts since the bot is always available, positive, and will never discuss. Patients may abuse the use of chatbots and can become addicted (Palanica et al. 2019). Here we need to find a balance between the desire of increasing adherence to therapy on the one hand and avoiding addiction and overreliance on the other hand.

Last but not least, we have to consider the technical limitations of chatbots in conjunction with their impact on people. In medicine, we recognize the current trend of personalization. A mental health chatbot personalizes responses and suggestions only to a certain extent. Aspects that are considered by therapists or physicians in treatment planning and decision making cannot be entirely be represented in a chatbot (even though AI is making advances in this respect). Therefore, mental health chatbots might be inappropriate for some patients, either due to the nature of their mental disorder (they might suggest help for people who cannot benefit from it) or due to personal preferences.

## 4.4   Accountability Implications

Mental health providers are accountable for providing competent care and maintaining patients' confidentiality due to the availability of laws and regulations that
protect patients' for any malpractice. In the case of chatbots, such liability is not available. In other words, there is a lack of laws and legislation that protect the privacy
and confidentiality of chatbot users. For instance, in the United States (where most
mental health chatbots were implemented), the Health Insurance and Portability and
Accountability Act (HIPAA) does not protect users' privacy of the majority of chatbots (Vaidyam et al. 2019). Furthermore, there is a lack of laws that protect chatbot
users when adverse events or undesirable outcomes happen (Palanica et al. 2019;
Whitby 2014). Although product liability laws may put some liability on chatbot
providers, they usually limit this liability by making no warranty and stating that chatbots do not provide professional therapy in the terms and conditions (Whitby 2014;
Martinez-Martin and Kreitmair 2018). This may legally protect chatbot providers.
First attempts towards a regulatory framework, through new legislation, are proposed
by Stiefel (Stiefel 2019). These attempts aim to limit the use and disclosure of
information received by software-based therapy technologies.

## 5   Future Research Directions

Application of AI-based chatbots for delivering mental healthcare provides several
benefits that were partially demonstrated by existing studies. Several open research
topics have to be addressed in future to create reliable mental health chatbots and to
integrate them into care processes.

   Among other things, there is still a need to improve the linguistic capabilities
of mental health chatbots (Laranjo et al. 2018). Their ability to understand and
to react appropriately to user input has to be increased. One big challenge is reliably detecting emergency situations and creating an appropriate reaction, once an
emergency situation has been detected. Customization or personalization of chatbots to individual users is another open issue (Kocaballi et al. 2019). Learning from
conversations with users could help. However, it is still an open question, whether
transferring knowledge from conversations and other data sources really results in
reliable chatbot systems or whether we lose control over system responses. Personalization also concerns considering the individual health literacy of a user. The style
or complexity of language could be adapted based on the given user input. Patient-
specific knowledge for example on treatment plans could be retrieved from health
records. Methods are required to include such knowledge dynamically to a chatbot.

   To ensure usage and usefulness, mental health chatbots have to be evaluated.
What are the relevant aspects for evaluating technical issues of healthcare chatbots?
Which criteria and metrics should be considered? If the evaluation of chatbots were
to align with practice of Evidence-Based Medicine (EBM) then the ideal is 'Level

1' evidence as produced by randomized controlled trials (RCTs). These trials are realised as summative evaluation to give electronic intervention credibility from an EBM perspective for selected health outcome measures. However, given the complex nature of a health chatbot and its potential interaction with users, we recommend use of a spectrum of quality measurements from across multiple dimensions that cover technical aspects, but also data security and efficiency to help ensure the feasibility and face-validity of the chatbot as the basis of a health intervention prior to attempting an RCT.

Researchers should pay more attention on how mental healthcare can derive benefits from the use of chatbots. Here, it will clearly be relevant to come up with new models of care that include chatbots in a way that the system reflects recommendations of the health carer and that it is aware of the treatment goals specified in the therapeutic session.

In conclusion, AI health chatbots are promising tools that could accompany a regular treatment in future. Before this can happen, many open issues and challenges still have to be addressed and more experiences in particular regarding negative aspects have to be gained.

# References

Abdul-Kader SA, Woods J (2015) Survey on chatbot design techniques in speech conversation systems. Int J Adv Comput Sci Appl 6(7). https://doi.org/10.14569/IJACSA.2015.060712

Anthes E (2016) Mental health: there's an app for that. Nature 532(7597):20–23

Abd-alrazaq AA, Alajlani M, Alalwan AA, Bewick BM, Gardner P, Househ M (2019) An overview of the features of chatbots in mental health: a scoping review. Int J Med Informatics 132:103978. https://doi.org/10.1016/j.ijmedinf.2019.103978

Abd-alrazaq AA, Alajlani M, Ali N, Denecke N, Bewickd BM, Househ M (2020a) Patients' attitudes toward using chatbots for mental health: scoping review. J Med Internet Res

Abd-alrazaq AA, Safi Z, Alajlani M, Warren J, Househ M, Denecke K (2020b) Technical metrics used to evaluate healthcare chatbots: scoping review. J Med Internet Res

Abd-alrazaq AA, Rababeh A, Alajlani M, Bewick BM, Househ M (2020c) The effectiveness and safety of using chatbots in mental health: a systematic review and meta-analysis

Bickmore TW, Caruso L, Clough-Gorr K, Heeren T (2005) 'It's just like you talk to a friend' relational agents for older adults. Interact Comput 17(6):711–735. https://doi.org/10.1016/j.int com.2005.09.002

Baer D (2016) What microsoft's teen chatbot being 'Tricked' into racism says about the internet. Business insider. https://www.businessinsider.com/what-microsoft-tay-says-about-the-internet-2016-3. Accessed 16 May 2020

Bendig E, Erb B, Schulze-Thuesing L, Baumeister H (2019) The next generation: chatbots in clinical psychology and psychotherapy to foster mental health—a scoping review. Verhaltenstherapie. https://doi.org/10.1159/000501812

Cuijpers P, Sijbrandij M, Koole SL, Andersson G, Beekman AT, Reynolds CF 3rd (2013) The efficacy of psychotherapy and pharmacotherapy in treating depressive and anxiety disorders: a meta-analysis of direct comparisons. World Psychiatry: Official J World Psychiatric Assoc (WPA) 12(2):137–148. https://doi.org/10.1002/wps.20038

Chung K, Park RC (2019) Chatbot-based heathcare service with a knowledge base for cloud computing. Clust Comput 22(1):1925–1937. https://doi.org/10.1007/s10586-018-2334-5

Csaky R (2019) Deep learning based chatbot models. arXiv preprint arXiv:190808835

Denecke K, Vaaheesan S, Arulnathan A (2020) Regulating emotions with the chatbot SERMO. IEEE Trans Emerg Topics Comput 1–13. https://doi.org/10.1109/TETC.2020.2974478

Fadhil A, Gabrielli S (2017) Addressing challenges in promoting healthy lifestyles: the al-chatbot approach. Paper presented at the proceedings of the 11th EAI international conference on pervasive computing technologies for healthcare, Barcelona, Spain

Fitzpatrick KK, Darcy A, Vierhile M (2017) Delivering cognitive behavior therapy to young adults with symptoms of depression and anxiety using a fully automated conversational agent (Woebot): a randomized controlled trial. JMIR Ment Health 4(2):e19. https://doi.org/10.2196/mental.7785

Fulmer R, Joerin A, Gentile B, Lakerink L, Rauws M (2018) Using psychological artificial intelligence (Tess) to relieve symptoms of depression and anxiety: randomized controlled trial. JMIR Ment Health 5(4):e64. https://doi.org/10.2196/mental.9782

Fiske A, Henningsen P, Buyx A (2019) Your robot therapist will see you now: ethical implications of embodied artificial intelligence in psychiatry, psychology, and psychotherapy. J Med Internet Res 21(5):e13216. https://doi.org/10.2196/13216

Grolleman J, van Dijk B, Nijholt A, van Emst A (2006) Break the habit! designing an e-therapy intervention using a virtual coach in aid of smoking cessation. In: International conference on persuasive technology. Springer, pp 133–141

Gao J, Galley M, Li L (2019) Neural approaches to conversational AI. Foundations and trends® in information retrieval 13(2–3):127–298. https://doi.org/10.1561/1500000074

Hester RD (2017) Lack of access to mental health services contributing to the high suicide rates among veterans. Int J Ment Heal Syst 11(1):47. https://doi.org/10.1186/s13033-017-0154-2

Hussain S, Ameri Sianaki O, Ababneh N (2019) A survey on conversational agents/Chatbots classification and design techniques. In: Cham. web, artificial intelligence and network applications. Springer International Publishing, pp 946–956

Inkster B, Sarda S, Subramanian V (2018) An empathy-driven, conversational artificial intelligence agent (Wysa) for digital mental well-being: real-world data evaluation mixed-methods study. JMIR Mhealth Uhealth 6(11):e12106. https://doi.org/10.2196/12106

Jurafsky D, Martin JH (2008) Speech and language processing: an introduction to speech recognition, computational linguistics and natural language processing. Prentice Hall Upper Saddle River, NJ

Jones SP, Patel V, Saxena S, Radcliffe N, Ali Al-Marri S, Darzi A (2014) How Google's 'Ten things we know to be true' could guide the development of mental health mobile apps. Health Affairs (project Hope) 33(9):1603–1611. https://doi.org/10.1377/hlthaff.2014.0380

Kocaballi AB, Berkovsky S, Quiroz JC, Laranjo L, Tong HL, Rezazadegan D, Briatore A, Coiera E (2019) The personalization of conversational agents in health care: systematic review. J Med Internet Res 21(11):e15360. https://doi.org/10.2196/15360

Kretzschmar K, Tyroll H, Pavarini G, Manzini A, Singh I (2019) Can your phone be your therapist? Young people's ethical perspectives on the use of fully automated conversational agents (Chatbots) in mental health support. Biomed Infor Insights 11:1178222619829083. https://doi.org/10.1177/1178222619829083

Lauzon FQ (2012) An introduction to deep learning. In: 2012 11th International conference on information science, signal processing and their applications (ISSPA). IEEE, pp 1438–1439

Luxton DD, Anderson SL, Anderson M (2016) Chapter 11—ethical issues and artificial intelligence technologies in behavioral and mental health care. In: Luxton DD (ed) Artificial intelligence in behavioral and mental health care. Academic Press, San Diego, pp 255–276. https://doi.org/10.1016/B978-0-12-420248-1.00011-8

Lucas GM, Rizzo A, Gratch J, Scherer S, Stratou G, Boberg J, Morency LP (2017) Reporting mental health symptoms: breaking down barriers to care with virtual human interviewers. Front Robot AI 4 (OCT). https://doi.org/10.3389/frobt.2017.00051

Laranjo L, Dunn AG, Tong HL, Kocaballi AB, Chen J, Bashir R, Surian D, Gallego B, Magrabi F, Lau AYS, Coiera E (2018) Conversational agents in healthcare: a systematic review. J Am Med Inform Assoc 25(9):1248–1258. https://doi.org/10.1093/jamia/ocy072

Lovejoy CA (2019) Technology and mental health: the role of artificial intelligence. Eur Psychiatry 55:1–3. https://doi.org/10.1016/j.eurpsy.2018.08.004

Luxton DD (2020) Ethical implications of conversational agents in global public health. Bull World Health Organ 98(4):285

Murray CJ, Vos T, Lozano R, Naghavi M, Flaxman AD, Michaud C, Ezzati M, Shibuya K, Salomon JA, Abdalla S et al (2012) Disability-adjusted life years (DALYs) for 291 diseases and injuries in 21 regions, 1990–2010: a systematic analysis for the global burden of disease study 2010. Lancet (london, England) 380(9859):2197–2223. https://doi.org/10.1016/s0140-6736(12)61689-4

Mental Health Foundation (2015) Fundamental facts about mental health. London

Martinez-Martin N, Kreitmair K (2018) Ethical issues for direct-to-consumer digital psychotherapy apps: addressing accountability, data protection, and consent. JMIR Ment Health 5(2):e32. https://doi.org/10.2196/mental.9423

Miller E, Polson D (2019) Apps, avatars, and robots: the future of mental healthcare. Issues Ment Health Nurs 40(3):208–214. https://doi.org/10.1080/01612840.2018.1524535

Nooijer JM, Oenema A, Kloek G, Brug J, De Vries H, De Vries NK (2005) Bevordering van gezond gedrag via Internet, nu en in de toekomst

Oladeji BD, Gureje O (2016) Brain drain: a challenge to global mental health. Bjpsych Int 13(3):61–63. https://doi.org/10.1192/s2056474000001240

Palanica A, Flaschner P, Thommandram A, Li M, Fossat Y (2019) Physicians' perceptions of chatbots in health care: cross-sectional web-based survey. J Med Internet Res 21(4):e12887. https://doi.org/10.2196/12887

Rahman AM, Mamun AA, Islam A (2017) Programming challenges of chatbot: current and future prospective. In: IEEE Region 10 humanitarian technology conference (R10-HTC), 21–23 Dec. 2017. pp 75–78. https://doi.org/10.1109/R10-HTC.2017.8288910

Shawar BA, Atwell ES (2005) Using corpora in machine-learning chatbot systems. Int J Corpus Linguist 10(4):489–516. https://doi.org/10.1075/ijcl.10.4.06sha

Sansonnet J-P, Leray D, Martin J-C (2006) Architecture of a framework for generic assisting conversational agents. In: Intelligent virtual agents. Springer Berlin Heidelberg, pp 145–156

Smith MJ, Ginger EJ, Wright M, Wright K, Humm LB, Olsen D, Bell MD, Fleming MF (2014) Virtual reality job interview training for individuals with psychiatric disabilities. J Nerv Ment Dis 202(9):659–667

Steel Z, Marnane C, Iranpour C, Chey T, Jackson JW, Patel V, Silove D (2014) The global prevalence of common mental disorders: a systematic review and meta-analysis 1980–2013. Int J Epidemiol 43(2):476–493. https://doi.org/10.1093/ije/dyu038

Stiefel S (2018) 'The chatbot will see you now': mental health confidentiality concerns in software therapy. https://doi.org/10.2139/ssrn.3166640

Stiefel S (2019) The chatbot will see you now: protecting mental health confidentiality in software applications. Sci Technol Law Rev 20(2). https://doi.org/10.7916/stlr.v20i2.4774

Tschanz M, Dorner TL, Holm J, Denecke K (2018) Using eMMA to manage medication. Computer 51(8):18–25. https://doi.org/10.1109/MC.2018.3191254

Torous J, Andersson G, Bertagnoli A, Christensen H, Cuijpers P, Firth J, Haim A, Hsin H, Hollis C, Lewis S, Mohr DC, Pratap A, Roux S, Sherrill J, Arean PA (2019) Towards a consensus around standards for smartphone apps and digital mental health. World Psychiatry: Official J World Psychiatric Assoc (WPA) 18(1):97–98. https://doi.org/10.1002/wps.20592

Ujiro T, Tanaka H, Adachi H, Kazui H, Ikeda M, Kudo T, Nakamura S (2018) Detection of dementia from responses to atypical questions asked by embodied conversational agents. Proc Interspeech 2018:1691–1695

Vaidyam AN, Wisniewski H, Halamka JD, Kashavan MS, Torous JB (2019) Chatbots and conversational agents in mental health: a review of the psychiatric landscape. Can J Psychiatry 0706743719828977

Weizenbaum J (1966) ELIZA—a computer program for the study of natural language communication between man and machine. Commun ACM 9(1):36–45. https://doi.org/10.1145/365153.365168

Whitby B (2014) The ethical implications of non-human agency in health care. In: Proceedings of MEMCA-14: (Machine ethics in the context of medical and care agents)

Whiteford HA, Ferrari AJ, Degenhardt L, Feigin V, Vos T (2015) The global burden of mental, neurological and substance use disorders: an analysis from the global burden of disease study 2010. PloS one 10(2):e0116820

Wilken B (2015) Methoden der Kognitiven Umstrukturierung: Ein Leitfaden für die psychotherapeutische Praxis" (Methods for cognitive restructuring—a guideline for psychotherapeutic practice). 8th edn. Kohlhammer Verlag

# AI and Machine Learning in Diabetes Management: Opportunity, Status, and Challenges

Marwa Qaraqe, Madhav Erraguntla, and Darpit Dave

**Abstract** Diabetes is a costly and burdensome metabolic disorder that occurs due to the elevated blood glucose levels. Poorly managed diabetes can lead to serious and life-threatening health complications. A person's glycated hemoglobin (HbA1C or A1C) measures the average blood glucose for the past 2–3 months by measuring how much glucose is bound to the hemoglobin cells in the blood. The HbA1C is used both to diagnose diabetes and assess the effectiveness of a person's management plan. Developing a model that can accurately predict a person's future HbA1C 2–3 months in advance holds immense potential for preventative and tailored medical care. With the new era of artificial intelligence (AI) it becomes increasing evident that some of unanswered health issues can be unlocked by leveraging on advanced AI and machine learning algorithms. In addition, sudden plummeted or elevated blood glucose levels also pose serious and life-threating consequences to diabetic people. The development of a detection and prediction model capable of detecting or predicting instances of hyperglycemia or hypoglycemia using new CGM technology is critical. This chapter discusses the consequences of poorly managed diabetes and how a more personalized treatment plan for diabetes may lie in the detection of hyper/hypoglycemic events and the prediction of a person's HbA1C using their current blood glucose values.

## 1 What is Diabetes?

Diabetes is a disorder that affects millions of people around the world. Diabetes impairs the body's ability to process blood glucose (blood sugar). The body breaks down the carbohydrates eaten into blood glucose which is then used to generate energy. Insulin is a hormone that the body needs to get glucose from the bloodstream into the cells of the body. Persons with diabetes are unable to produce insulin or do

M. Qaraqe (✉) · M. Erraguntla · D. Dave
Division of Information and Computing Technology, Hamad Bin Khalifa University, Doha, Qatar
e-mail: mqaraqe@hbku.edu.qa

© Springer Nature Switzerland AG 2021                                                    129
M. Househ et al. (eds.), *Multiple Perspectives on Artificial Intelligence in Healthcare*,
Lecture Notes in Bioengineering, https://doi.org/10.1007/978-3-030-67303-1_11

not use it efficiently. Without careful management, diabetes can lead to a buildup of sugars in the blood, increasing the risk of serious complications, including stroke, heart disease, vision impairment, and infection.

## 1.1 Forms of Diabetes

For Type 1 diabetes, the exact cause is still unclear to doctors, but genetics and environmental aspects seem to play an important role. In this form of diabetes, the body produces little to no insulin, thereby requiring patients to use insulin therapy and other treatments to manage their condition.

Type 2 diabetes has a stronger link to family history and lineage than type 1, but it also depends on environmental and lifestyle factors. Type 2 patients still produce insulin, but the receptors at the cell are unable to capture the glucose from the blood stream. Insulin allows the glucose from a person's food to access the cells in their body to supply energy.

In the case of type 2 diabetes, insulin resistance takes place gradually. Leading a healthy and active lifestyle and eating well-balanced meals can help in delaying or offsetting the development of type 2 diabetes.

Gestational diabetes occurs in pregnant women due to their body becoming less sensitive to the insulin produced. This form of diabetes does not occur in all pregnant woman and usually is resolved after delivery. However, women who develop gestation diabetes are at increased risk in developing type 2 diabetes later.

## 1.2 Diagnosis

There are several ways that doctors diagnose diabetes. The first and most infamous is called the glycated hemoglobin (HbA1C or A1C) test. This test measures the average blood glucose for the past 2–3 months by measuring how much glucose is bound to the hemoglobin in the blood. This testing method does not require fasting or drinking a sugary solution. An A1C of greater than or equal to 6.5% indicates diabetes. Table highlights A1C levels and their corresponding diagnosis.

The fasting plasma glucose (FPG) test checks the fasting blood glucose levels. Fasting blood glucose levels of greater than or equal to 126 mg/dl indicates a high probability of diabetes. Table 1 shows the normal, prediabetes range, and diabetes FPG range. Another test that is commonly used by physicians in the diagnosis of diabetes, particularly for gestational diabetes, is the oral glucose tolerance test (OGTT). This test is a two-hour long test that requires patients to drink a special sugary drink when fasting. Blood glucose levels are checked prior to drinking the solution, one hour after, and two hour after consumption. This test enables doctors

**Table 1** Hemoglobin A1C, FPG, and OGGT levels and corresponding diagnosis

| Diagnosis | HbA1C (%) | FPG (mg/dl) | OGTT (mg/dl) |
| --- | --- | --- | --- |
| Normal | Less than 5.7 | Less than 100 | Less than 14 |
| Prediabetes | 5.7–6.4 | 100–125 | 140–199 |
| Diabetes | 6.5 or higher | 126 or higher | 200 or higher |

to assess how the body processes glucose. A two hour blood glucose of great than or equal to 200 mg/dl indicates diabetes. The diagnostic range of the OGTT test is listed in Table 1.

## 2 Importance of Diabetes Management

Diabetes is a disorder that requires constant management. In addition to medication, self-management of diabetes is very important to prevent acute complications and minimize the risk of long-term complications. Management of diabetes includes efficiently inducing self-care behaviors among the patients, such as scheduling meals, counting carbohydrates intake, monitoring daily blood glucose trends, exercising, and tracking aim-oriented life behaviors on a daily basis. Nonadherence to any of the aforementioned activities may lead to lead to long-term complications such as heart disease, stroke, blindness, amputation, kidney disease, dental disease, and increased susceptibility to infections (Diabetes Prevention Program Research Group, op.cit.; CDC, National Diabetes Statistic Report 2017). As a consequence, diabetes management becomes a cumbersome and complex task, and should account for diverse factors, such as medications, personal behaviors, and life-related activities. These factors must be jointly be optimized in order to improve the quality of life a person with diabetes.

### 2.1 Retinopathy and Blindness

Uncontrolled blood glucose levels, over time, can cause damage to small blood vessels within the retina of the eye. This damage can cause vision loss by two common ways: (1) a disease known as proliferative retinopathy, and (2) macular oedema. Proliferative retinopathy occurs when weak and abnormal blood vessels develop on the surface of the retina and leak fluids onto the center of the eye. Macular oedema occurs when fluid leaks from the blood vessels into the center of the macula causing it to swell. If left untreated, people with diabetic retinopathy can potentially lose vision in the eye affected. Figure 1 shows the results of a study by CDC, National Diabetes Statistic Report (2017) that concludes that diabetes is the leading cause of

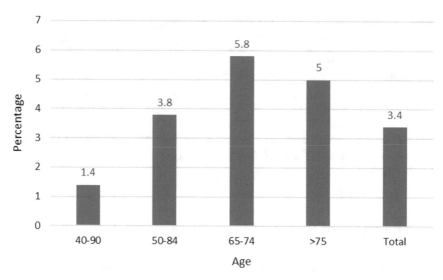

**Fig. 1** Prevalence of diabetic retinopathy among adults 40 years or older (CDC, National Diabetes Statistic Report 2017)

new cases of blindness among young adults (aged 20–74) where 12,000–24,000 new cases of blindness each year is reported due to diabetic retinopathy.

## 2.2 Kidney Disease

Long term high blood glucose levels also have damaging effects on the kidneys. In particular, uncontrolled blood glucose increases the risk of developing diabetic nephropathy. This disease begins long before any symptoms appear and slowly damages parts of the kidney that is responsible for filtering the blood. Left untreated, this disease can cause total kidney failure, requiring patients to undergo dialysis treatment. In the United States, diabetes is the leading cause for kidney failure accounting for 43% of new cases each year (NIDDK 2004).

## 2.3 Heart Disease and High Blood Pressure

Diabetes and heart disease are intricately connected. People with diabetes may have several underlying conditions, such as high blood pressure, high cholesterol, and obesity, which increases their risk for heart disease. Managing their blood glucose levels greatly decreases the risk of the development of heart disease. The prevalence of high blood pressure in diabetic people is approximately 73%. In addition, adults with diabetes have four times increased risk for heart disease related death than adults without diabetes, and these statistics are predicted to increase in the upcoming years. Due to the link between poor management of diabetes and heart disease, it is imperative to take courses of actions to properly monitor and manage glucose levels (Diabetes Prevention Program Research Group, op.cit.).

## 2.4 Other Diabetes Associated Diseases

Along with the aforementioned diabetes related diseases, approximately 60–70% of diabetes patients suffer from mild to severe forms of nervous system damage (Diabetes Prevention Program Research Group, op.cit.). Long term high blood glucose levels often cause impaired sensations or pain the feet and hands, sometime causing amputation of lower-extremity limbs. In particular, in the US alone, 60% of non-trauma related lower-limb amputations are among persons with diabetes. Approximately 82,000 lower-limb amputations were performed among persons with diabetes just between the years 2000–2001 (CDC, National Diabetes Statistic Report 2017).

In general, people with uncontrolled diabetes have higher risks to develop other diseases. They are also more susceptible to have longer recovery times or worse symptoms from other illnesses such as the flu or pneumonia. Thus, it is evident that proper management of the disease is imperative to live a healthy and normal life.

## 2.5 Effective Management Technologies

Continuous Glucose Monitoring (CGM) is a method to track glucose observations at regular intervals (typically every few minutes) throughout the day (Hess 2019). CGM devices have a sensor that is inserted under the skin that measures glucose values. Typically a CGM device is composed of two main components:

(a) Sensor: The sensor is a small wire that is inserted under the skin which measures the interstitial glucose levels from the subcutaneous tissue space.

(b) Transmitter: The transmitter captures the readings from the sensor. This information is then transmitted wirelessly to an attached insulin pump device or a separate device like a reader or a phone via near field communication (NFC) or Bluetooth.

The development of these CGM devices revolutionized diabetes self-management. Traditional methods of using a manual fingerstick to measure blood glucose only provides a "snapshot" of the glucose level at a point in time, whereas, CGM devices allow better visibility of the glucose trends as the readings are continuously measured. As a consequence, it benefits the patient in gaining insight about their glucose trends throughout the day and helps them optimize their food intake and plan physical

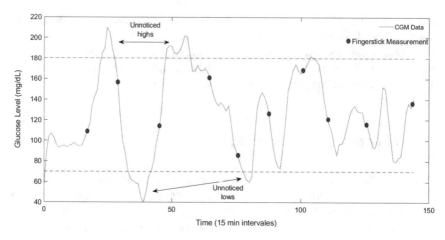

**Fig. 2** CGM plot illustrating benefits of CGM over periodic fingerstick glucose measurements

activity. With full access to a patient's glucose trends, clinicians can prescribe a better treatment plan/therapy for a patient in Fig. 2 shows the benefits of analyzing CGM data versus traditional methods. In the figure, the fingerstick measures not only do not give a good representation of the patient's glucose trend, they fail to capture critical instances when the patient's blood glucose was above and below safe levels.

CGM devices have allowed patients to achieve good glycemic control and reduce glycemic excursion (fluctuations in blood sugar), thereby decreasing both hypoglycemia (low glucose) and hyperglycemia (high glucose) instances (Rodbard 2017). Modern-day CGM devices come with an inbuilt functionality that provides notifications if the glucose readings are reaching or are likely to reach below specified thresholds in the imminent future. This helps patients take preventative measures to avoid serious outcomes. In addition, CGM devices present opportunities for in-depth analysis to be performed on the data that is being captured. With the advancement of ML and AI methodologies, valuable insights on factors influencing glucose levels can be extracted and provide critical functionalities for improving patient care. The next section highlights how CGM data has been exploited using AI methods.

## 3 The Integration of AI and Machine Learning for Diabetes Care

The AI methodologies used in the area of health management in general and diabetes management in particular can be divided into two broad categories, namely, expert systems and machine learning. An expert system (ES) represents one of most common types of AI which assists care givers in their routine work by capturing expert knowledge, facts and reasoning techniques. The aim is to mimic clinician's expertise to support decision making. In the area of diabetes, the most common

ES used are rule-based reasoning (RBR), case-based reasoning (CBR) and fuzzy systems. RBR is based on transferring the knowledge of an expert to a computer in the form of conditions and rules, while CBR uses previous experience to find solutions to new problems similar to previously seen examples. However, fuzzy systems generally translate expert knowledge and account for ambiguity and degrees in class assignment. For instance, typically a blood glucose range <70 mg/dl is considered low and >180 mg/dl is considered high. However, this definition does not accommodate finer distinctions within low and high classes. A high value of 185 mg/dl is clinically different than 285 mg/dl and both cannot be simply classified in the same 'High' class. In fuzzy modeling, 185 mg/dl is high but can be acceptable, while 285 mg/dl can never be acceptable.

Machine learning (ML) is the ability of a machine to learn over time without being explicitly programmed. In the medical field, ML algorithms are extensively used to extract valuable knowledge from large databases, such as medical records. Methods of ML that are extensively applied in the field of diabetes management include, but limited to, decision trees (DT), support vector machines (SVM), artificial neural networks (ANN), genetic algorithms (GA), and deep learning. There has been significant work in the literature that leverage on ML methods for the prediction and management of diabetes. The work in Yu et al. (2010) implemented SVM to test its ability to classify individuals with diabetes mellitus. The authors of Lopez et al. (2018) used the random forest (RF) algorithm to select corresponding attributes single-nucleotide polymorphism (SNPs) responsible for diabetes mellitus. A modified LR model for detecting the most relevant predictor of T2DM was investigated in Devi et al. (2016). The work in Mhaskar et al. (2017) proposed a deep neural network-based approach for blood glucose monitoring. They used a semi-supervised method with three networks of the different clusters and a final layer to predict the output. Their model achieved accuracies of accuracies of 88.72% (hypoglycemia), 80.32% (euglycemia) and 64.88% (hyperglycemia). Because early detection or prediction of diabetes is important in its prevention or proper management, research has recently focused on using the power of AI for predicting diabetes (Barakat et al. 2010; Zhang et al. 2017; Xu et al. 2017; Malik et al. 2016; Thulasi et al. 2017; Alghamdi et al. 2017; Heikes et al. 2008; Stern et al. 2002; Abdul-Ghani et al. 2007, 2011; Tripathy et al. 2000) using a variety of clinical data, ranging from images to blood plasma levels.

## 3.1 Estimated HbA1C Versus Predictive HbA1C

The HbA1C is considered the "gold-standard" when it comes to diagnosing and managing diabetes. HbA1C is based on a laboratory test from a blood sample to measure the accumulated blood glucose over a 2–3-month span. As mentioned in Sect. 2, consistently elevated blood glucose levels cause a variety of health issues. The future prediction of the HbA1C based on the CGM data holds a critical significance in maintaining long term health of diabetes patients. There has been significant work done on conversion formulas that estimate HbA1C using past average blood glucose levels. In particular, research from a clinical study, Diabetes Control and Complications Trial (DCCT)), derived the mathematical formula, $eHbA1C = \frac{AG+77.3}{35.6}$ as an appropriate estimate for laboratory tested HbA1C measures, where AG denotes the average blood glucose level. Variations for the estimated HbA1C have been proposed throughout the literature, however, the aforementioned mathematical models only provide instantaneous estimated HbA1C levels of past blood glucose and provide no information on future values. In order to assess whether a patient's current medical treatment and lifestyle plan is appropriate, predictions of HbA1C based on current trends is needed.

### 3.1.1 Challenges of HbA1C Prediction

Long-term predictive HbA1C measures using short-term CGM data is a revolutionary idea but is yet to be achieved due to the complexity of the problem. Although AI methods have evolved dramatically in the past decade, HbA1C prediction using only CGM data is still challenging even for the most robust AI techniques as the data provided (7–14 days of CGM data) is transient and is subject to various external influences/ interventions. In particular, three main challenges are identified when it comes to HbA1C prediction based on CGM readings, namely, (1) data samples over a short time duration, (2) highly varying nature of the data, and (3) missing data. The CGM sensors in the market usually measure blood glucose every 5–15 min thus generating 96–288 measurements per day. Occasionally, patients might remove sensors due to certain events or sensors might become dislodged and stop collecting data. This presents large time spans of missing blood glucose measurements. Developing algorithms that can accurately estimate missing blood glucose values is a challenge and usually suffer from high error rates. Ignoring the missing data creates misleading blood glucose trends and negatively affects the prediction accuracy.

Blood glucose measurements are highly variable and depend on a number of factors such as erythropoiesis (iron and vitamin B12 deficiency, liver disease, etc.) and altered hemoglobin glycation (alcoholism, renal failure, aspirin, vitamin C and E, etc.). Consequently, devising an accurate HbA1C prediction algorithm is difficult if a patient's full health history and lifestyle choices are not incorporated into the algorithm, but generally integrating such information is difficult and not-realistic. In addition, two patients may have similar HbA1C measures but their CGM trends may be drastically different. This phenomenon creates a "many-to-one" scenario where varying CGM trends can potentially equate to similar HbA1C measures, increasing the difficulty of accurate predictions.

The prediction of HbA1C thus boils down to extracting optimized features from CGM data and integrating these features with state-of-the-art AI techniques for prediction. Due to the increasing popularity of CGM sensors and improvements in data analytics field, this gap in research will soon be filled.

## 3.2 CGM Based Hyper and Hypoglycemia Predictions

### 3.2.1 Prediction and Challenges

Predicting a hypoglycemic (low glucose) and hyperglycemic (high glucose) at least 30–60 min in advance provides enough time for a patient to take corrective measures. The challenge of predicting impending episodes with high true positive rates (sensitivity) and high true negative rates (specificity) remains a key issue for patients and clinicians. Addressing this challenge could be a landmark achievement in the treatment of diabetic patients as it would lead to saving of many lives. Many of the existing alarm functionalities are plagued with giving too many "false alerts". As a result, patients are inclined to turn-off notifications, which defeats the purpose of the alerts. A typical patient is out of normal range only 1–10% of the time. The uneven class membership makes development of AI and Machine learning capabilities for accurate predictions difficult (Hu et al. 2009). Contextual information such as physical activity, sleep, driving, and food intake all have an effect on blood glucose values (Allen and Gupta 2019; Rodbard 2016) but relevant data is unavailable in real-time. Although devices such as wearables and Smartphone Apps are available to capture most of these data, integrated data is not currently available to facilitate real-time glucose predictions.

### 3.2.2 Current Literature

Researchers have tried to solve the glucose prediction problem using two main approaches:

(a) regression-based approach: Predicting the exact glucose value into the future
(b) classification-based approach: Predicting a probabilistic estimate of the risk of low or high glucose levels at a future time point.

Existing literature for CGM prediction has generally looked into a prediction horizon between 15 and 60 min, giving ample time for a patient to take corrective measures. The first professional CGM device was approved by the United States F.D.A. in 1999. Since then, many studies have been published in the diabetes literature about the prediction of glucose levels. The earlier methods relied more on classical statistical modelling such as Autoregressive Integrated Moving Average (ARIMA), linear regression, etc., but as machine learning became more popular and accessible, researchers adopted sophisticated machine learning algorithms like Random Forests, Support Vector Machines, Boosting, Neural Networks for addressing this prediction problem. The work in Gadaleta (2018) provides a summary of the different methodologies used in this application area.

Despite the progress made, there are some fundamental issues that need to be tackled to facilitate practical, robust, and universal AI and ML based solution to this serious health problem:

**Table 2** Sample RMSE results for various glycemic ranges

| CGM range | Reported RMSE | Glycemic state |
|---|---|---|
| <55 | 20.12 | Severe hypoglycemia |
| ≥55 and <70 | 15.75 | Hypoglycemia |
| ≥70 and <80 | 1.08 | Normal range |
| ≥180 and <300 | 15.87 | Hyperglycemia |
| ≥300 | 18.8 | Severe hyperglycemia |
| Overall results | 6.65 | |

(a) Standard data: Results reported in the literature have been obtained through analysis on different datasets. Some studies have relied on simulated data (Cappon 2018; Dassau 2010; Li, et al. 2019; Mahmoudi 2014; Reddy, et al. 2019; Zecchin 2012), UVA/ Padova Type 1 Diabetes simulator being the more popular, for obtaining data for analysis. Some studies have also collected data through a controlled pilot, where data is collected from patients through camps ranging from a few hours to few days. Only a handful of the existing studies have based their results on data collected from subjects in real-world settings. Being human specific, a lot of influencing factors such as age, gender, glycemic profile, lifestyle, etc. determine the glucose variability within a patient's body. Because of the relatively small data volumes, performance of machine learning algorithms are highly dependent on the dataset used. In the absence of standard datasets, it becomes difficult to unbiasedly evaluate different approaches in the literature. A large, open and standardized data that researchers can use to objectively test and evaluate performance of algorithms will be helpful to address this need.

(b) Standard comparison metrics: The most widely used metrics for reporting regression results is the root-mean-squared error (RMSE) which is the square root of the mean of squares of differences between the predicted and actual CGM values. However, it will be critical to evaluate the RMSE of the results in different target ranges. For example, in Table 2, though the overall RMSE is very low, a deeper look into the results among various glycemic ranges will show that the particular method doesn't work too well for prediction in lower and higher ranges which are more important to diabetes control. Due to higher number of observations in the normal range, the overall RMSE appears to be misleadingly low. There is a need to evaluate RMSE in critical glucose ranges for effective diabetes management.

In the classification approaches, due to the presence of imbalanced classes, it is required to evaluate performance using both sensitivity and specificity or alternately both precision and recall. Some studies report only one of these metrics or use non-standard metrics such as "number of false alarms per week" (Dassau 2010). There is a need to use standard classifier evaluation criterion such as sensitivity and specificity to compare different AI and ML approaches.

(c) Hypoglycemic/ Hyperglycemic definition: Majority of the studies in the literature consider a CGM reading less than 70 mg/dL as a hypoglycemic event and a reading above 200 mg/dL as hyperglycemic, but there are instances where a different criterion is used. Some studies (Cameron 2008; Georga 2013; Jensen 2013, 2014) need more than 2 consecutive readings below a threshold to define a hypoglycemic/hyperglycemic event, and a few other studies combine all the readings within a time window below the threshold value as a single hypoglycemic/hyperglycemic event. Such variations make it difficult to evaluate different approaches in the literature.

# 4 Long Term Unmet Challenges

Technological advancements have been very beneficial to patients with diabetes—be it measuring glucose levels in real-time or the predictive capabilities incorporated in these devices, patients are being benefitted in improving their overall glycemic profile. However, there are some areas that need critical improvements. Firstly, though glucose observations are available in real-time, currently data related to insulin delivery from insulin pumps is not available in real-time. Especially for Type 1 diabetes patients, the CGM devices are often used in association with insulin pump (Pettus and Edelman 2017) which injects insulin at preset times or at user initiated times during a day (insulin bolus). Secondly, food intake and its macronutrient breakdown, especially carbohydrates have a substantial impact on glucose levels. Many Smartphone applications are available on different platforms for tracking a person's food intake and calculating the associated nutrition value for different food items. But integrated datasets covering CGM and food intake are currently not available. Physical activity is another important factor influencing blood glucose values. With the plethora of fitness devices available today, measuring physical activity with good accuracy isn't a hurdle anymore, but integrated CGM and physical activity data are also not available. There is a need to perform clinical studies to facilitate collection of CGM and associated contextual data (sleep, food intake, insulin intake, and physical activity) to facilitate next generation AI and ML solutions.

# 5 Future Work

Significant progress has been made in the CGM technology in regards to the device accuracy and predictive capabilities of AI/ML algorithms (Dave et al. 2019). These have been very beneficial to clinicians and patients. We believe that, the next round of innovations would come in addressing some of the challenges we discussed earlier. Especially integrating contextual information will help catapult existing predictive models for primetime usage and position them to better address diabetes management. Though most patients with type 1 diabetes use insulin pump in conjunction with the CGM device, the necessary settings to inject insulin are currently preset and doesn't change dynamically based on real-time glucose readings. Integrated AI and ML based analysis of CGM, insulin pump, and contextual data will result in dynamic calibration of insulin to meet real-time needs of the patient, thus achieving the vision of artificial pancreas (Allen and Gupta 2019).

# References

Abdul-Ghani MA, Williams K, DeFronzo RA, Stern M (2007) What is the best predictor of future type 2 diabetes? Diabetes Care 30(6):1544–1548

Abdul-Ghani MA, Abdul-Ghani T, P. Stern M, Karavic J, Tuomi T, Bo I, DeFronzo RA, Groop L (2011) Two-step approach for the prediction of future type 2 diabetes risk. Diabetes Care p DC 102201

Alghamdi M, Al-Mallah M, Keteyian S, Brawner C, Ehrman J, Sakr S (2017) Predicting diabetes mellitus using smote and ensemble machine learning approach: the henry ford exercise testing (fit) project. PloS one 12(7):e0179805

Allen N, Gupta A (2019) Current diabetes technology: striving for the artificial pancreas. Diagnostics 9(1):31

Barakat N, Bradley AP, Barakat MNH (2010) Intelligible support vector machines for diagnosis of diabetes mellitus. IEEE Trans Inf Technol Biomed 14(4):1114–1120

Cameron F et al (2008) Statistical hypoglycemia prediction. J Diabetes Sci Technol 2(4):612–621

Cappon G et al (2018) A neural-network-based approach to personalize insulin bolus calculation using continuous glucose monitoring. J Diabetes Sci Technol 12(2):265–272

CDC (2017) National Diabetes Statistic Report

Dassau E et al (2010) Real-time hypoglycemia prediction suite using continuous glucose monitoring: a safety net for the artificial pancreas. Diabetes Care 33(6):1249–1254

Dave D et al (2019) Feature selection based machine learning algorithm for real-time hypoglycemia prediction. T.A.M. University, Hospital TCS, Medicine BCO (eds) J Biomed Health Inf (JBHI) Submitted: 16 Sep 2019

Devi MN, Balamurugan AA, Kris MR (2016) Developing a modified logistic regression model for diabetes mellitus and identifying the important factors of type ii dm. Indian J Sci Technol 9(4)

Diabetes Prevention Research Group, op.cit.

Gadaleta M et al (2018) Prediction of adverse glycemic events from continuous glucose monitoring signal. IEEE J Biomed Health Inform 23(2):650–659

Georga EI et al (2013) A glucose model based on support vector regression for the prediction of hypoglycemic events under free-living conditions. Diabetes Technol Ther 15(8):634–643

Heikes KE, Eddy DM, Arondekar B, Schlessinger L (2008) Diabetes Risk Calculator: a simple tool for detecting undiagnosed diabetes and prediabetes. Diabetes Care 31(5):1040–1045

Hess A (2019) What is a Continuous Glucose Monitor (CGM)? Available from: https://www.ontrackdiabetes.com/type-1-diabetes/what-continuous-glucose-monitor-cgm. Accessed 15 Aug 2019

Hu S et al (2009) MSMOTE: improving classification performance when training data is imbalanced. In: 2009 second international workshop on computer science and engineering, IEEE

Jensen MH et al (2013) Real-time hypoglycemia detection from continuous glucose monitoring data of subjects with type 1 diabetes. Diabetes Technol Ther 15(7):538–543

Jensen MH et al (2014) Evaluation of an algorithm for retrospective hypoglycemia detection using professional continuous glucose monitoring data. J Diabetes Sci Technol 8(1):117–122

Lopez BL, Torrent-Fontbona F, Vinas R, Fernandez-Real JM (2018) Single nucleotide polymorphism relevance learning with random forests for type 2 diabetes risk prediction. Artif intell med 85:43–49

Li K et al (2019) GluNet: a deep learning framework for accurate glucose forecasting. IEEE J Biomed Health Inf 24(2):414–423

Mahmoudi Z et al (2014) Accuracy evaluation of a new real-time continuous glucose monitoring algorithm in hypoglycemia. Diabetes Technol Ther 16(10):667–678

Malik S, Khadgawat R, Anand S, Gupta S (2016) Non-invasive detection of fasting blood glucose level via electrochemical measurement of saliva. Springerplus 5(1):701

Mhaskar HN, Pereverzyev SV, van der Walt MD (2017) A deep learning approach to diabetic blood glucose prediction. Front Appl Math Stat 3:14

National Institute of Diabetes and Digestive and Kidney Diseases (NIDDK) (2004) National diabetes statistics. NIH Publication No. 04–3892. Available at: http://diabetes.niddk.nih.gov/dm/pubs/statistics/index.htm

Nai-arun N, Moungmai R (2015) Comparison of classifiers for the risk of diabetes prediction. Procedia Computer Science 69:132–142

Pettus J, Edelman SV (2017) Recommendations for using real-time continuous glucose monitoring (rtCGM) data for insulin adjustments in type 1 diabetes. J Diabetes Sci Technol 11(1):138–147

Reddy R et al. (2019) Prediction of hypoglycemia during aerobic exercise in adults with type 1 diabetes. Journal of Diabetes Science and Technology 13(5):919–927

Rodbard D (2016) Continuous glucose monitoring: a review of successes, challenges, and opportunities. Diabetes Technol Ther 18(S2):S2-3–S2-13

Rodbard D (2017) Continuous glucose monitoring: a review of recent studies demonstrating improved glycemic outcomes. Diabetes Technol Ther 19(S3):S-25–S-37

Stern MP, Williams K, Haffner SM (2002) Identification of persons at high risk for type 2 diabetes mellitus: do we need the oral glucose tolerance test? Ann Intern Med 136(8):575–581

Thulasi K, Ninu E, Shiva KK (2017) Classification of diabetic patients records using naïve bayes classifier. In: 2017 2nd IEEE international conference on recent trends in electronics, information & communication technology (RTEICT), IEEE, pp 1194–1198

Tripathy D, Carlsson M, Almgren P, Isomaa B, Taskinen M-R, Tuomi T, Groop LC (2000) Insulin secretion and insulin sensitivity in relation to glucose tolerance: lessons from the Botnia study. Diabetes 49(6):975–980

Xu W, Zhang J, Zhang Q, Wei X (2017) Risk prediction of type ii diabetes based on random forest model. In: 2017 Third international conference on advances in electrical, electronics, information, communication and bio-informatics (AEEICB), IEEE, pp 382–386

Yu W, Liu T, Valdez R, Gwinn M, Khoury MJ (2010) Application of support vector machine modeling for prediction of common diseases: the case of diabetes and pre-diabetes. BMC Med Inform Decis Mak 10(1):16

Zecchin C et al (2012) Neural network incorporating meal information improves accuracy of short-time prediction of glucose concentration. IEEE Trans Biomed Eng 59(6):1550–1560

Zhang J, Xu J, Hu X, Chen Q, Tu L, Huang J, Cui J (2017) Diagnostic method of diabetes based on support vector machine and tongue images. BioMed Res Int 2017

# AI From a Technological Perspective

# Reinforcement Learning Applications in Health Informatics

**Abdulrahman Takiddin, Mohamed Elhissi, Salman Abuhaliqa, and Yin Yang**

**Abstract** Reinforcement learning (RL) is a branch of Artificial intelligence (AI) that makes complex decisions all by itself. Unlike traditional AI systems that passively absorb knowledge provided by humans, the RL technology actively teaches itself through trial and error by interacting with a simulated environment. RL is used in various domains including video games, robotics, natural language processing, and financial analysis. This chapter discusses the opportunities that RL provides in the healthcare field, along with the challenges and limitations associated with each of its applications. Specifically, the adoption of RL in the Internet of Things healthcare devices, medication dosing, drug design, treatment recommendation, lung radiotherapy, personal health, and sepsis treatment has overcome a number of challenges. For example, RL helps in determining the dosage for patients, designing drugs, and guiding patients towards a healthier lifestyle. However, the use of RL in the healthcare field is still limited by the availability and accuracy of relevant medical datasets, requires further validation, and takes time to adapt to changes in the environment.

**Keywords** Reinforcement learning · Artificial intelligence · Healthcare IoT · Therapy · Medication

## 1 Introduction

Recent years have witnessed a renaissance of artificial intelligent (AI) technologies, powered by deep neural networks, which promise to revolutionize healthcare by automating key processes traditionally performed by human doctors. Among the new wave of AI techniques, reinforcement learning (RL) is a particularly promising methodology, in which *the AI makes complex decisions all by itself* (e.g., on treatment plans (Wang et al. 2018), medication dosage (Nemati et al. 2016), drug design

A. Takiddin · M. Elhissi · S. Abuhaliqa · Y. Yang (✉)
College of Science and Engineering, Hamad Bin Khalifa University, Doha, Qatar
e-mail: yyang@hbku.edu.qa

A. Takiddin
e-mail: atakiddin@hbku.edu.qa

© Springer Nature Switzerland AG 2021
M. Househ et al. (eds.), *Multiple Perspectives on Artificial Intelligence in Healthcare*,
Lecture Notes in Bioengineering, https://doi.org/10.1007/978-3-030-67303-1_12

(Stahl et al. 2019), etc.), instead of merely providing information to the human doctor. Further, unlike traditional AI systems that passively absorb knowledge provided by humans, in RL, *the AI actively teaches itself* through trial and error by interacting with a simulated environment.

To design a new drug, for example, an RL AI agent neither blindly enumerates possible drug designs in a brute-force fashion (as traditional search-based AI systems do), nor learns purely from a massive pile of past drug design records (as most machine-learning-based AI systems do). Instead, the AI aims to discover an effective *policy* for designing new drugs. To do so, the AI starts from a basic policy of randomly generating organic molecules and iteratively improves itself by (i) applying its current policy to create new drugs and (ii) observing the effectiveness of the created drugs (as *reward signals*) and learning from the *experience* of observations and rewards as guidance to improve its design policy. The fact that the AI actively *explores* the design space in Step (i) above means that it may identify new strategies never attempted before by human experts. Meanwhile, through the learning step in Step (ii), the AI improves its policy by *exploiting* its past experience, which allows it to navigate a vast search space efficiently, in an educated manner.

Due to the above characteristics (i.e., extensive and efficient explorations of the policy space), RL promises to outperform humans in decision making. This already happened in competitive board games (Silver et al. 2018) and computer games (Berner et al. 1912). In particular, the AI agent has demonstrated the ability to conceive and apply complex strategies that achieve *long-term benefits*, e.g., sacrificing a piece in a chess game for an advantageous position many moves later (Silver et al. 2018). Further, the AI also learns to *co-operate* with other agents, e.g., by sacrificing its own health points to cover up for a team member in a war game (Berner et al. 1912).

Besides learning through trial and error, an RL agent can also directly learn from human experiences, e.g., summarized in past patient treatment records and outcomes of a certain type of disease (Wang et al. 2018). Essentially, this combines RL and traditional supervised learning. Finally, RL is also commonly applied as a *meta-learning* technique, which identifies an effective policy to learn from data. For instance, the state of the art in image recognition (e.g., diagnosing diseases from X-ray images) employs RL to design the structure of the convolutional neural network (Elsken et al. 1808) as well as the algorithm to augment input images (Cubuk et al. 2019).

In the following, we elaborate on the concept of RL in Sect. 2, and its promising applications in healthcare in Sect. 3. In Sect. 4, we summarize the findings, and we make the conclusions in Sect. 5.

## 2 Reinforcement Learning

RL is a machine learning (ML) framework that is used for obtaining the optimum output from an environment based on the information obtained while performing trial and error (Notsu et al. 2018). Unlike the other ML frameworks, supervised learning and unsupervised learning, in RL, labeled input and output pairs are not needed. Also, sub-optimal actions do not have to be explicitly corrected. Instead, RL focuses on finding the balance between exploring the uncharted space and the current knowledge (Sutton and Barto 2018).

RL can be used when actions are chosen at a time-step based on their current state. Then, the agent receives the evaluative feedback and the new state from the environment. This iterative process stops until the goal of the optimal policy is reached. The optimal policy is achieved when the accumulated reward it receives over time is maximized. In an RL environment, no direct instructions on the actions that should be taken are provided, instead they are learned through the trial and error interactions with the environment. This process is called adaptive closed-loop feature, which distinguishes RL from the traditional supervised learning methods where the list of correct labels has to be provided and from unsupervised learning approaches, where some reduction in the dimensionality or density estimation has to occur (Littman 2015). Moreover, RL develops a control policy directly from the experience to predict states and rewards during the learning process, unlike the traditional techniques where a mathematical model of the environment is required.

The aforementioned features make RL a better approach when it comes to efficiency, representation, and generalization, theoretically and technically (Li 2018), which led to an increase of RL applications in many real-life environments. For example, RL has been used in video games, self-driving, robotics, natural language processing, art creation, business management, and financial analysis (Notsu et al. 2018). Additionally, RL has been used in biological analysis and healthcare systems (Yu et al. 1908).

## 3 Reinforcement Learning in Healthcare

RL has been used in many healthcare domains, especially that the decision-making process of medical treatment is based on a sequential procedure. For example, the treatment is based on the treatment type, drug dosage, re-examination timing, and the current health status and the treatment history of a patient (Yu et al. 1908). Currently, these decisions are made using randomized controlled trials that derive from the average population response. However, if RL is used, the medical decisions will be personalized for each patient that might have high heterogeneity in response to the treatment due to the variety in disease severity, personal characteristics, and drug sensitivity. RL is able to find optimal policies using only previous experiences, without requiring any prior knowledge about the mathematical model of the biological systems. These aspects make RL more appealing than the existing control-based or randomized approaches in healthcare domains. It is almost impossible to build an accurate model that would accommodate the variety of responses of treatment and interactions in human bodies (Yu et al. 1908).

The rest of the chapter focuses on the use of RL in the healthcare domain, including the Internet of Things (IoT), medication dosing, drug design, treatment recommendation, lung radiotherapy, personal health, and sepsis treatment. Each subsection discusses the solutions that RL offers along with the associated limitations.

## 3.1   Healthcare IoT

IoT refers to any object or service that is connected to a network at any time in any place (Islam et al. 2015). IoT has made its way to play a significant role in healthcare since it is capable of sending or sharing medical information from the medical devices to any other device that is connected to the internet. For example, IoT is used in remote health monitoring, fitness applications, and elderly care to send alarms or notifications in case of emergency (Min et al. 2018).

Healthcare IoT devices can use the energy harvesting (EH) technique, which is using the energy from the environment, such as the ambient radio frequency and the body motion to extend the battery life. Herein, RL is used as a privacy-aware offloading scheme for the EH powered healthcare IoT devices. RL can learn to select the offloading and local computing rates without knowing the privacy leakage, IoT energy consumption, and edge computation model. This is used in evaluating the privacy level, energy consumption, and computation latency to choose the offloading policy to the edge device in each time slot. This is used to achieve the optimal offloading policy by performing iterative trial-and-error using the learning method model that makes use of the IoT offloading experiences and builds an architecture to generate simulated experiences while the value function of the RL technique is being updated literately (Min et al. 2018). However, the use of RL in IoT devices is limited since RL algorithms will not be capable of handling changes in sensors and actuators. Also, the trained RL algorithm will require a significant training time in case the number of devices or sensors increased.

## 3.2   Medication Dosing

Determining the actual needed quantity and the dosage of medicine varies from one patient to another. RL is used for the medication dosing given the sequential nature of the medical treatment, where multiple treatment decisions are performed without being aware of the actual effectiveness of each stage as there is no clear match between the actions and outcomes of each dosage. Therefore, identifying the dosage with the positive effect from the negative one is challenging. Additionally, medical intentions can be misleading when it comes to predicting the effects of a sequence of treatments over time. RL aims to solve those uncertainties as it learns, for each patient, the dosing policy and maximizes the overall fraction of time given all aspects about the patients, including their therapeutic activated partial thromboplastin time (aPTT) range (Nemati et al. 2016). Despite the benefits that RL offers in determining the medication dosage, such a technique is limited by the availability of extensive medical granular temporal data, which are often deficient (Nemati et al. 2016).

## 3.3   Drug Design

New drug discovery can result from a de novo design, where a well-motivated hypothesis for new lead compound generation is used, or from compound selection using available or synthetically feasible chemical libraries based on the readily available structure-activity relationship (SAR) data (Schnecke and Bostrom 2006). However, both methods come with challenges. The de novo design drug hypotheses are understandably biased toward preferred chemistry or driven by model interpretation. The diversity of the synthetically feasible chemicals using SAR data, that may be considered a potential drug-like molecule, is estimated to be between $10^{30}$ and $10^{60}$, which prohibits the systematic exploration of all of these possibilities (Polishchuk et al. 2013).

Different methods have been proposed to tackle these challenges. The first method includes the local optimization approaches that are optimized either by stochastic sampling or restricting the search to a defined chemical space that result in loss of likely significant possibilities (Reker and Schneider 2015). The second method is the chemical space exploration based on continuous encoding of molecules. This method was efficient, but it did not provide weight towards special physical or biological properties (Gómez-Bombarelli et al. 2018). The third method includes the generation of focused molecular libraries using recurrent neural networks (RNNs), which could not control the molecular properties of the produced molecules (Segler et al. 2018).

In addition to the aforementioned attempts, a novel method that uses RL to generate compounds with desired physical, chemical, and bioactivity properties was offered as a plausible solution that minimized the deficiencies of the previously discussed techniques (Popova et al. 2018). The main innovative aspect of this approach includes the simple representation of molecules by the simplified molecular-input line-entry system (SMILES) strings only for both generative and predictive phases of the method. Then, it integrates these phases into a single workflow that includes an RL module (Popova et al. 2018). The result of this work was promising to produce a de novo drug design with the desired physiochemical and biological properties. However, there is a limitation associated with this approach as it is incapable of affording multi-objective optimization of multiple target properties simultaneously. This is required when the molecules of a particular drug have to be optimized, given the drug-likeness properties.

## 3.4  Treatment Recommendation

The use of supervised RL along with an RNN (SRL-RNN) is employed for treatment strategy recommendation. This method combines the indicator signal and evaluation signal to discover the optimal treatment. It also provides the patient with a dynamic treatment regime (Wang et al. 2018). The SRL-RNN model is trained on doctors' historical prescription data and demonstrated that it is capable of reducing the estimated mortality rates and providing better medication recommendation as well (Wang et al. 2018). However, the accuracy of such an approach depends on the accuracy of the doctors' historical prescription data that the model is trained on. Also, it depends on the availability of relevant prescription data for new patients that react differently to treatments.

## 3.5  Lung Radiotherapy

There are two major subtypes of lung cancer, namely, small cell lung cancer (SCLC) and non-small cell lung cancer (NSCLC) (Jaffray 2012). Since NSCLC is generally in-operable, the cornerstone of management is radiation therapy (radiotherapy) (Jaffray 2012). Despite the significant advances in the technologies of radiotherapy planning, the treatment outcomes are generally not promising (Jaffray 2012), and it has been postulated that the escalation of the radiation dose may improve the disease outcomes (Eisbruch et al. 2017). However, meticulous measures should be taken to balance the benefits, mainly expressed in terms of local control (LC) with the risk factors, mainly radiation-induced pneumonitis (RP), which may significantly decrease the patient's quality of life. The famous RTOG-0617 clinical trial results, where dose escalation has led to surprisingly negative results, concluded that dose escalation could not be employed using a one-size-fits-all approach to the patient population (Bradley et al. 2015).

Using retrospective treatment plans for patient with NSCLC, HH (Tseng et al. 2017) investigated the use of RL to develop automated radiation adaptation protocols for NSCLC that aims to maximize the tumor local control at the reduced rates of radiation-induced pneumonitis. A neural network framework that contains three components is used for RL for dose fractionation adaptation. In addition to lung and tumor dosimetric variables, multiple patient characteristics were used, including clinical, genetics, and imaging radiomics features. The aforementioned RL model is able to provide dosing recommendations that are similar to the clinician's recommendations although the dataset is small. This carries promising potentials to optimize personalized radiotherapy dosages with the least side-effects. On the other hand, this framework requires further validation using more datasets. Additionally, this framework considers a single adaptation action of changing the dosage instead of formulating an adaptation protocol that is continuous (e.g., on a daily or weekly basis) (Tseng et al. 2017).

## 3.6  Personal Health Advisor

According to the World Health Organization, an unhealthy lifestyle represents the highest cause of death (Chen et al. 2018). The utilization of RL is to inform users about their unhealthy behaviors and guide them accordingly (Chen et al. 2018). By using the smart personal health advisor (SPHA), successful guidance can be provided to the patient. The proposed system uses a multidimensional health data to monitor patient health (Chen et al. 2018). An SPHA-Score is used, which denotes a healthy lifestyle by monitoring both physiological and psychological user data. Using this SPHA-Score model and utilizing RL provides an intelligent and successful health monitoring and guidance system. Considering that the multidimensional multi-modal data collected by sensors provides a dynamic evaluation standard, RL is employed to determine the best strategy for maximum cumulative reward (Chen et al. 2018). However, when major changes in patients' lifestyles take place, it would take the proposed RL-based system a considerable amount of time to adapt itself to those changes. As a result, the RL-based system might provide inaccurate recommendations during transition periods.

## 3.7  Sepsis Treatment

Sepsis treatment is highly challenging since every patient reacts differently to treatment and no standard treatment method for sepsis is being used (Raghu et al. 2017). The use of RL to deduce treatment policies is employed in sepsis treatment to find a better strategy for patient treatment (Raghu et al. 2017). Unlike the traditional approach, the RL-based approach is data-driven. By modeling the state of a patient and his/her physiological data in the intensive care unit, RL is employed to find the suitable set of actions and learn treatment policies. This way, the patient's treatments and wellbeing outcomes are improved. As a result, patient mortality rates are reduced. In order to keep the reward function for the RL clinically sound, two measures are used to indicate the overall patient health, including the sequential organ failure assessment (SOFA) and the lactate level, which is a measure of cell-hypoxia that is usually higher in septic patients (Raghu et al. 2017). However, to prove that, further improvements in the quantitative analysis has to be done since statistical guarantees of the performance are not provided.

## 4  Summary

Table 1 summarizes the challenges that RL overcomes, the opportunities it offers, and the limitations associated with each of the aforementioned applications of RL in healthcare. Employing RL in the healthcare IoT devices helps reduce energy

**Table 1** Summary of findings

| Application | Challenges | Opportunities | Limitations |
|---|---|---|---|
| Healthcare IoT (Min et al. 2018) | High energy consumption and privacy leakage in healthcare IoT devices | Used as a privacy-aware offloading scheme for energy harvesting powered healthcare IoT devices | Incapability of handling changes in the IoT devices |
| Medication dosing (Nemati et al. 2016) | Identifying the positive and negative effect of a specific dosage | Determines the quantity and dosage of medicines with their effects | Availability of large detailed clinical datasets |
| Drug design (Popova et al. 2018) | Designing a drug is biased towards preferred chemistry | Generates drugs with desired properties without bias | Incapability of affording multi-objective optimization of multiple target properties |
| Treatment recommendation (Wang et al. 2018) | Finding the optimal prescription for the patient | Handles complex relations among multiple medications, diseases and individual characteristics | Depends on the accuracy of doctors' historical prescription data |
| Lung radiotherapy (Tseng et al. 2017) | Radiation cannot be employed using a one-size-fits-all approach to all patients | Maximizes the tumor control at the reduced rates of radiation | Requires further validation using more datasets |
| Personal health advisor (Chen et al. 2018) | General health guidelines for all users | Informs users about unhealthy behaviors and guides them accordingly | Adapting to major changes takes time |
| Sepsis treatment (Raghu et al. 2017) | Finding a personalized treatment method per patient | Provides the optimal strategy for patient treatment | Needs further statistical proofs |

consumption, but it is incapable of handling changes in the states of the IoT device. RL is also used to determine the quantity and dosage of medicines, but it is subject to the availability of large detailed clinical datasets. To overcome the bias towards the preferred chemistry, RL helps generate drugs with desired properties without bias, but it is incapable of affording multi-objective optimization of multiple target properties. Using RL along with RNN helps find the optimal prescription for patients using doctors' historical prescription data. Hence, the accuracy of such an approach is tied to the accuracy of doctors' datasets. To overcome the issue of using a standard radiation approach for all patients, RL is employed to maximize the tumor control at the reduced rates of radiation, but further validation is still required. Instead of providing generalized health guidelines, RL provides user-specific guidelines based on the user's behavior, but it takes time to adapt itself to major lifestyle changes. RL offers the optimal patient-specific strategy treatment, but further studies are needed to statistically prove its significance.

# 5 Conclusion

Reinforcement learning (RL) is being used in different domains, including healthcare. Specifically, the adoption of RL in the Internet of Things healthcare devices, medication dosing, drug design, treatment recommendation, lung radiotherapy, personal health, and sepsis treatment has overcome a number of challenges. For example, RL helps in determining the dosage for patients, designing drugs, and guides patients towards a healthier lifestyle. However, using RL in the healthcare field is limited by the availability and accuracy of relevant medical datasets, requires further validation, and takes time to adapt to changes.

# References

Berner C, Brockman G, Chan B, Cheung V, Debiak P, Dennison C, Farhi D, Fischer Q, Hashme S, Hesse C et al (2019) Dota 2 with large scale deep reinforcement learning. arXiv preprint arXiv: 1912.06680

Bradley JD, Paulus R, Komaki R, Masters G, Blumenschein G, Schild S, Bogart J, Hu C, Forster K, Magliocco A et al (2015) Standarddose versus high-dose conformal radiotherapy with concurrent and consolidation carboplatin plus paclitaxel with or without cetuximab for patients with stage IIIA or IIIB non-small-cell lung cancer (RTOG 0617): a randomised, two-by-two factorial phase 3 study. Lancet Oncol 16(2):187–199

Chen M, Zhang Y, Qiu M, Guizani N, Hao Y (2018) SPHA: smart personal health advisor based on deep analytics. IEEE Commun Mag 56(3):164–169

Cubuk ED, Zoph B, Mane D, Vasudevan V, Le QV (2019) Autoaugment: learning augmentation strategies from data. In: Proceedings of the IEEE conference on computer vision and pattern recognition, pp 113–123

Eisbruch A, Lawrence TS, Pan C, Ten Haken RK, Frey K, Arenberg D, Moran J, Cease K, Orringer M, Curtis J et al (2017) Using FDG-PET acquired during the course of radiation therapy to individualize adaptive radiation dose escalation in patients with non-small cell lung cancer

Elsken T, Metzen JH, Hutter F (2018) Neural architecture search: a survey. arXiv preprint arXiv: 1808.05377

Gómez-Bombarelli R, Wei JN, Duvenaud D, Hernández-Lobato JM, Sánchez-Lengeling B, Sheberla D, Aguilera-Iparraguirre J, Hirzel TD, Adams RP, Aspuru-Guzik A (2018) Automatic chemical design using a data-driven continuous representation of molecules. ACS Cent Sci 4(2):268–276

Islam SR, Kwak D, Kabir MH, Hossain M, Kwak K-S (2015) The internet of things for health care: a comprehensive survey. IEEE Access 3:678–708

Jaffray DA (2012) Image-guided radiotherapy: from current concept to future perspectives. Nat Rev Clin Oncol 9(12):688

Li Y (2018) Deep reinforcement learning. CoRR abs/1810.06339 [Online]. Available: http://arxiv. org/abs/1810.06339

Littman ML (2015) Reinforcement learning improves behaviour from evaluative feedback. Nature 521(7553):445–451

Min M, Wan X, Xiao L, Chen Y, Xia M, Wu D, Dai H (2018) Learning-based privacy-aware offloading for healthcare IoT with energy harvesting. IEEE Internet Things J 6(3):4307–4316

Nemati S, Ghassemi MM, Clifford GD (2016) Optimal medication dosing from suboptimal clinical examples: a deep reinforcement learning approach. In: 2016 38th Annual international conference of the IEEE engineering in medicine and biology society (EMBC). IEEE, pp 2978–2981

Notsu A, Yasuda K, Ubukata S, Honda K (2018) Optimization of learning cycles in online reinforcement learning systems. In: 2018 IEEE international conference on systems, man, and cybernetics (SMC). IEEE, pp 3530–3534

Polishchuk PG, Madzhidov TI, Varnek A (2013) Estimation of the size of drug-like chemical space based on gdb-17 data. J Comput Aided Mol Des 27(8):675–679

Popova M, Isayev O, Tropsha A (2018) Deep reinforcement learning for de novo drug design. Sci Adv 4(7):eaap7885

Raghu A, Komorowski M, Ahmed I, Celi L, Szolovits P, Ghassemi M (2017) Deep reinforcement learning for sepsis treatment. arXiv preprint arXiv:1711.09602

Reker D, Schneider G (2015) Active-learning strategies in computerassisted drug discovery. Drug Discovery Today 20(4):458–465

Schnecke V, Bostrom J (2006) Computational chemistry-driven decision making in lead generation. Drug Discovery Today 11(1–2):43–50

Segler MH, Kogej T, Tyrchan C, Waller MP (2018) Generating focused molecule libraries for drug discovery with recurrent neural networks. ACS Cent Sci 4(1):120–131

Silver D, Hubert T, Schrittwieser J, Antonoglou I, Lai M, Guez A, Lanctot M, Sifre L, Kumaran D, Graepel T et al (2018) A general reinforcement learning algorithm that masters chess, shogi, and go through self-play. Science 362(6419):1140–1144

Stahl N, Falkman G, Karlsson A, Mathiason G, Bostrom J (2019) Deep reinforcement learning for multiparameter optimization in de novo drug design. J Chem Inf Model 59(7):3166–3176

Sutton RS, Barto AG (2018) Reinforcement learning: an introduction. MIT Press

Tseng H-H, Luo Y, Cui S, Chien J-T, Ten Haken RK, El Naqa I (2017) Deep reinforcement learning for automated radiation adaptation in lung cancer. Med Phys 44(12):6690–6705

Wang L, Zhang W, He X, Zha H (2018) Supervised reinforcement learning with recurrent neural network for dynamic treatment recommendation. In: Proceedings of the 24th ACM SIGKDD international conference on knowledge discovery & data mining, 2018, pp 2447–2456

Yu C, Liu J, Nemati S (2019) Reinforcement learning in healthcare: a survey. arXiv preprint arXiv: 1908.08796

# Deep Learning in Healthcare

**Samir Brahim Belhaouari and Ashhadul Islam**

**Abstract** Artificial Intelligence (AI) and Deep Learning (DL) have been household names in research in the past decade. This chapter discusses the application of deep learning on healthcare, specifically in detection of cancer. It enumerates the state-of-art research work on lungs, liver, breast and brain cancer and then focuses on the scope of deep learning in healthcare, discussing some of the emerging areas of research. The chapter also touches upon the limitations of using deep learning as a standard vehicle of diagnostics in healthcare. As there is little doubt that the Deep Learning methods will find a strong foothold in the healthcare domain, this chapter elucidates the tenets of Deep Learning to data science practitioners and healthcare workers alike so that these methods can be better used for the welfare of life on Earth.

## 1  Deep Learning—An Overview

Artificial Intelligence (AI) is a branch of science that studies ways to build intelligent programs and machines that can solve problems on their own. It is defined in the leading textbooks as the study of "intelligent agents": a device that is capable of understanding its environment and then takes actions that enhance its probability of achieving the goals. (Poole et al. 1998) Machine Learning (ML) is a subsection of AI that enables systems with the ability to automatically improve from experience. (Mitchell 1997) ML consists of algorithms that are designed to build a mathematical model based on data provided. Without being explicitly programmed, they learn from the data and make predictions or decisions. (Koza et al. 1996) Deep Learning (DL) is one step further into the foray of learning from experience. It is part of the family of

**Electronic supplementary material** The online version of this chapter
(https://doi.org/10.1007/978-3-030-67303-1_13) contains supplementary material, which is available to authorized users.

S. B. Belhaouari (✉) · A. Islam
Division of Information and Communication Technologies, Hamad Bin Khalifa University, Doha, Qatar
e-mail: sbelhaouari@hbku.edu.qa

M. Househ et al. (eds.), *Multiple Perspectives on Artificial Intelligence in Healthcare*,
Lecture Notes in Bioengineering, https://doi.org/10.1007/978-3-030-67303-1_13

machine learning methods; however, it is inspired from the structure of arrangement of neurons in the animal brain (Kleene 1956).

The rapid expansion of big data and the advances of hardware systems have boosted the popularity of Deep Learning among researchers and practitioners alike. Advancing from the earlier rule-based AI systems, Deep Learning today involves creating expert systems by learning from labelled data. The model (network) for a pre-defined task (e.g. breast cancer detection from mammography) is trained using labeled training inputs and the corresponding categories they belong to (example infected or non-infected). The trained model then can be used to predict the possible label for a new unlabeled data set (mammogram image). The advantage of deep learning lies in the fact that it can autonomously teach itself data-directed, well represented hierarchical features and as a result perform extraction of feature and classification on a network without human intervention. Unlike before, the onus of deriving features no longer lies on the human, but the network can, by itself, derive features that make sense to the network and derive surprisingly accurate results. Deep Learning is thus, especially useful in assisting the physicians by enhancing the clinical diagnostic process. These intelligent systems increase the efficiency of decisions, making them more effective by reducing errors, thereby elevating patient safety and reducing costs. This chapter presents different methods and technologies of Deep Learning, the contemporary areas of research, the scope and the limitations. The chapter also takes cancer detection as a case study and elaborates the use of Deep Learning in the same.

Deep learning has ushered in a new era in the domain of research. It has found its application in different fields, among which the field of health informatics has seen promising advancements over the last few years. There are no doubts about the benefits of artificially intelligent systems in healthcare. They take into consideration several attributes of patients' data, including the differences in molecular traits, diagnostic medical images, related environmental factors, electronic health records and lifestyle. Researchers train intelligent models to learn how clinicians respond to patient details and diagnostic images. These models are then able to identify outcomes of tests, analyze treatment responses and predict susceptibility to diseases or chances of re admission. Deep learning comes with many advantages like the fact that it can be trained on unlabeled data. It is also capable of handling complex and multi-dimensional data internally and independently. Inspired by neural networks, these Deep Learning algorithms employ techniques to generate weights, extract high-level features and information without any manual intervention. This results in generation of more objective and unbiased classification results. The giant strides taken by the Deep Learning research domain would not have been possible without the adequate processing support provided by Graphical Processing Units or GPUs and Tensor Processing Units or TPUs. As a result, plenty of experimental work have implemented deep learning models for health informatics, creating alternative techniques that have been used by many technicians. In this context, the health team of DeepMind, an Artificial Intelligence company, in collaboration with Moorfields Eye Hospital NHS Foundation Trust is working on detecting eye disease from scans as accurately as experts (Fauw et al. 2018). The team has also worked with University

College London Hospitals NHS Foundation Trust on planning cancer radiotherapy treatment (Nikolov et al. 2018). There is no doubt that Deep Learning is going to play a pivotal role in revolutionizing health care and pave the way for newer innovations that will help humanity at large.

## 2   Scope of Deep Learning in Healthcare

One of the fields which is thought to be most suitable to be profoundly impacted by AI tools and techniques is the healthcare field. Some of the common application of traditional machine learning in healthcare is precision medicine—predicting which treatment procedures are likely to succeed on a patient based on the condition of the patient and the treatment context (Lee et al. 2018). Mandatory practices such as Electronic Medical Records ensure that such patient data is made available for the models to train on. AI and Machine Learning enhance the quality of intelligent decision-making in patient care and public health systems to transform the lives of billions around the world. We will now go through some key examples of modern applications of AI/DL in healthcare.

## 2.1   Cancer Diagnosis

Magnetic resonance imaging or MRI and other advanced medical imaging techniques are armed with Deep Learning algorithms that are increasingly forming the first level of checks for cancer detection. As the number and quality of radiologists are unable to meet up with the overwhelming digitized data coming out of these imaging systems, deep learning-based systems are useful in assisting the decision-making process. We shall discuss this in detail in the following sections.

### AI Assistance in Radiology and Pathology

The deluge of medical data puts trained radiologists under enormous strain. An average radiologist has to go through one image every 3–4 s in an 8-h workday to meet the workload expectations (Hosny and Chintan 2018).

There is no dearth of imaging data and DL algorithms can be fed with the ever-expanding dataset of the same to find patterns and interpret the results in the same way that a highly trained radiologist would. The algorithms can be taught the difference between benign and abnormal results, identifying suspicious characteristics in the images. These algorithms are more useful in identifying rare or difficult to diagnose diseases. Being trained on large datasets containing images of these diseases, they are often more dependable than humans when it comes to detecting edge-cases. This has been implemented by Microsoft in its Project InnerEye (Microsoft 2016) which utilizes machine learning to differentiate between tumors and healthy anatomy using

3 Dimensional radiological images that help medical experts in radiotherapy and surgical planning.

**AI in Actionable Medical Insights**

With the increasing amount of digitized patient record, there is a need to connect to a multitude of databases and analyze a mixture of radiology images, blood reports, Electrocardiograms or ECGs, genomics, patient medical history and others. Not only this, systems should be able to project their analysis and patterns discovered into human readable form so that doctors and healthcare professionals can work on these results to prescribe affordable and responsible diagnosis. One example of such fruitful collaboration between machine and radiologists can be found at Enlitic, a San Francisco based start-up. (Lyman, https://www.enlitic.com/) Not only do they couple world-class radiologists with data scientists and engineers, they also claim to analyze the world's most comprehensive clinical data, creating medical software that allow doctors to diagnose quickly with greater accuracy.

**AI for Healthcare Operation Management**

Long queue, fear of getting unreasonable bills, frustrating appointment process, not getting paired up with the right professional are some of the reasons why visiting healthcare facilities has become a daunting task. AI and other data-driven techniques can handle these issues and thereby smoothen the operational issues in a healthcare system. AI techniques can be used to create solutions of these problems as these kinds of pattern matching and optimization problems are best solved using large databases and intelligent search algorithms which are strengths of AI. As more patients pro-actively participate in their own well-being, the outcomes improve—resources are utilized better, financial outcomes and stakeholder experience are enriched. The goal is to develop and deploy suitable AI-assisted platforms whose main objective is to enhance the experience of healthcare services for people in general. Businesses in other sectors have employed such large-scale AI solutions to improve their operational efficiency. The difference between these businesses and healthcare is that, while AI systems in general businesses try to maximize profit, the AI tools in healthcare balance the goal of profit generation with the aspect of empathy.

Let us now elaborate on the application of Deep Learning in Cancer detection.

## 3   Deep Learning and Cancer

### 3.1   The Threat of Cancer

According to the World Health Organization, cancer is the second leading causes of death all over the world and was responsible for 9.6 million deaths in 2018 (WHO 2021). Not only is it a lethal affliction, it is painful because of the ordeal that a person diagnosed with cancer has to go through. The chemotherapy, for many, is a distressing process with many side effects that cause the patients to feel awkward and alienated.

The chances of recovery for a patient at a late stage of cancer is quite bleak. On a global scale, almost 1 in 6 deaths is the result of cancer and the prevalent types are cancers of Lung, Liver, Colorectal, Stomach and Breast (WHO 2021). Moreover, it has been seen that around 70% of deaths from cancer happen in countries having low and mid-level incomes (WHO 2021).

It is alarming to note that more than 14 million new cases of cancer are reported every year and it is expected that over the next two decades, the number of new cases will rise by 70% (Exchange 2017).

## 3.2 Cancer Diagnosis and Deep Learning

Early detection is one of the most important criteria to curb the ill effects of cancer. When it comes to diagnosis of the disease, the role of the human examiner is of paramount importance. Traditionally, decisions are made based on the physician's memory and judgement of the symptoms and ailments. However, the limited extent of human memory and the rapidly increasing knowledge base creates the need for developing computing tools that will help humans in the decision-making process.

In order to make the process of cancer diagnosis faster and more accurate, machines have been assisting doctors and pathologists since the early 1980s (Doi 2007). A computer can do thousands of biopsies in a few seconds. It can repeat itself thousands of time without exhaustion and get better with every repetition. Humans too get better with practice; however, the human endurance lies nowhere close to that of a machine. With the advent of Internet-Of-Things (IOT) and the ubiquitous presence of data, machines have a vast ocean of datasets to learn from and consequently machines have become very good at finding patterns and predicting results.

In the early stages of cancer, it is never easy to detect the discrepancies. Manual interpretation of medical images require time, effort and a trained eye. It is also highly prone to mistakes. This is where Deep Learning systems can help by bringing in key insights from the vast knowledge base on which they are modelled.

In the following sections we summarize the different deep learning methods employed in the detection of cancer in lungs, breast, brain and liver.

## 3.3 Deep Learning in Lung Cancer Detection

As can be seen in Fig. 1, lung cancer is on the top of mortality list compared to other cancer types (WHO 2021). This makes it a threat and a big challenge in the medical field.

Several types of deep learning architectures are introduced by various researchers in order to classify lung cancer. We will describe a few of the notable ones.

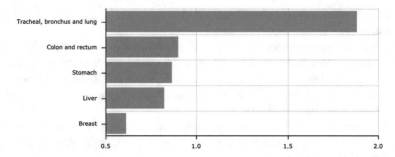

**Fig. 1** Death rate by cancer type in 2018 in millions for all ages and both sexes

## *3.4 Google Research on Lung Cancer Detection*

Google research team have shown that a deep learning tool can be used to detect lung cancer with high accuracy (Ardila et al. 2019). The team developed a model using 45,856 de-identified chest computerized tomography (CT) screening cases from National Institute of Health's National Lung Screening Trial study and North-Western University. The model was then compared with 6 board certified radiologists. When using a single CT scan for diagnosis, the model performed at par or outperformed the human radiologists. AUC of the algorithm was 94.4% and the model improved both on false positives as well as false negatives. The model has the additional feature of detecting inconspicuous malignant tissues in the lungs. Moreover, it brings into consideration data from previous scans and often identifies temporal growth of suspicious tissues that indicates malignancy.

## *3.5 Detecting Cancer with Double Convolutional Network*

This method was developed by training a double convoluted neural network using CT scans. (Jakimovski and Davcev 2019). The CT images were acquired from the Image & Data Archive of the University of South Carolina and the Laboratory of Neuro Imaging (LONI) database (Carolina 2021). The retrieved images were analysed and classified as cancerous or not by medical personnel after performing a biopsy of the lung cancer tissue. This made sure that the labelling was correctly performed.

The researchers employed a double Convolutional Deep Neural Network (CDNN) on different stages of lung cancer to determine the stage at which the double CDNN was able to detect the possibility of lung cancer. After extensive training over 100 epochs, the double CDNN model achieved an accuracy of 0.9962. The researchers claim that using this algorithm, the doctors will have help in early identification and treatment of lung cancer (Jakimovski and Davcev 2019).

## 3.6 Deep Learning in Breast Cancer Detection

Breast cancer is the most common form of cancer among women, affecting around 2.1 million women each year. In 2018, around 627,000 women died from breast cancer—that is approximately 15% of all cancer deaths among women (Omar et al. 2020).

The most commonly used technique for early detection of cancer is Mammography (Tariq 2018). The medical practitioners examine mammograms and recommend biopsy if abnormalities are found in the mammogram. Although biopsy is a standard clinical approach used to detect breast cancer, it is a costly, time consuming and painful process. In case of incorrect diagnosis, patients have to go through unnecessary biopsy (Jalalian et al. 2017). In order to help the radiologist improve their accuracy, Machine Learning and AI can play a critical role.

The idea behind using ML in breast cancer detection is based on training a model on a set of mammogram images. Different researches have proved the efficiency of ML methods and different feature extraction techniques for the detection of breast cancer. Below is a brief review of some related works on cancer detection and malignancy classification those have shown promising results (Fig. 2).

Eltoukhy et al. (2010) have presented a texture extraction method based on curvelet transform that is proved to be efficient with smooth objects. The authors used MIAS dataset to classify benign and malignant tumours. The classification accuracy achieved is 97.03%.

Zheng et al. (2018) have proposed a CNN classification model that is based on a VGG-19 pre-trained network. They have made use of cascading features using three detectors (Haar, LBP, and HOG). The classification distinguishes between cancerous and non-cancerous tissues. The model has results in a specificity of 0.991.

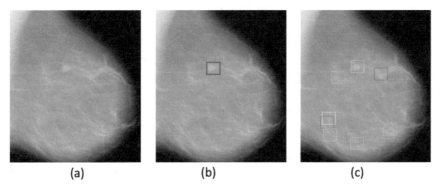

(a)  (b)  (c)

**Fig. 2** Mammogram image (**a**), detection of suspicious tissues (**b**), and abnormality localization (**c**) (Eltoukhy et al. 2010)

## 3.7 Deep Learning in Brain Cancer Detection

Early diagnosis of brain cancer plays a major role in the treatment of cancer. Machine learning methods are used to enhance brain cancer diagnosis using MRI images. In this type of cancer, the available data is much less than other types, which makes the task more challenging. Usually in DNN, transfer learning is used to achieve good results. Transfer learning is using a pre-trained network and tunes its hyperparameters by using the available dataset. Following are some research work done on detection of Brain cancer using deep learning.

Sobhaninia et al. (2019) tackles the segmentation of brain tumour using images from different angles and views. The authors state that a single network does not achieve accurate segmentation in all views. Hence, they have proposed classifying the image view and then training different networks for different views. The F1 score for this experiment was 78%.

Table 1 shows a summarized view of different types of cancer and the relevant research work performed on those areas. The first column defines the type of cancer in focus. The second column gives the details about the authors and the year in which the work was published. The third column enumerates the datasets used in the research while the fourth one defines the method of classification that was used in the work.

To understand the performance of the methods proposed the accuracy of the models have been mentioned in the last column. In a binary classification problem, the accuracy is usually measured as the total number of correct classifications divided by the total number of classifications.

The confusion matrix is a very useful tool in understanding the overall efficiency of any classifier. It is expressed as follows.

$$Confusion\ matrix = \begin{bmatrix} True\ Positive(TP) & False\ Positive(FP) \\ False\ Negative(FN) & True\ Negative(TN) \end{bmatrix}$$

True Positive(TP) is the number of cases correctly identified while False Positive is the number of datapoints that are not afflicted but the model identifies them to be afflicted.

False Negative(FN) is the number of cases that are actually afflicted and yet the model classifies them as not afflicted. True Negative(TN) on the other hand is the number of cases that are correctly identified as not affected.

The confusion matrix leads to some more measures of accuracy.

**Sensitivity or Recall** is the ratio between how many values were correctly classified as positive and how many were truly positive.

**Specificity** is the ratio between how many values were correctly classified as negative to how many were actually negative.

**Precision** measures out of all positive cases, how many were correctly classified as positive.

**Table 1** Summary of existing work of different types of cancer

| Cancer Type | Author, year and reference number | Dataset | Classification method | Accuracy |
|---|---|---|---|---|
| Lung cancer | Alakwaa et al. (2017) | Kaggle CT scan (Booz and Hamilton (2017)) | Convoluted neural network(CNN) | 86.6% |
| | (Hosny et al. 2018) | HarvardRT Radboud Maastro Moffitt MUMC M-SPORE RIDER (Hosny, https://journals. plos.org/plosmedic ine/article?id=10. 1371/journal.pmed. 1002711) | CNN | 99% |
| | (Xu et al. 2019) | 268 patients CT scans (Xu et al. 2019) | Combined CNN and Recurrent neural network (RNN) | – |
| Breast cancer | Eltoukhy et al. (2010) Zheng et al. (2018) | MIAS (Mammographic Image Analysis Homepage 2021) | K nearest neighbours (KNN) | 97.03% |
| | Tariq (2017) Jalalian et al. (2017) | Mini-MIAS (Suckling 2021) | Artificial neural network (ANN) | 99.1–100% |
| | Zheng et al. (2018) Sobhaninia et al. (2019) | UCHC DigiMammo (UConn 2021) | CNN | Specificity: 0.991 |
| | (Le et al. 2019) | SEER (National cancer institute, https://seer.cancer. gov/) (Le 2020) | CNN | 89% |
| | (Wu et al. 2019) | Cameylon 16 (CAMELYON16 2021) (Medgift 2021) | Combined CNN and RNN | 85% |

(continued)

**F1 score** is the harmonic mean of precision and recall and is a measure of the model's classification ability.

**Table 1** (continued)

| Cancer Type | Author, year and reference number | Dataset | Classification method | Accuracy |
|---|---|---|---|---|
| Liver cancer | Ginneken et al. (2019) | LiTS (Christ 2021) | CNN | 77% |
| | Das et al. (2019) | LiTS (Christ 2021) | Deep Neural Network (DNN) | 99.38% |
| | (Gruber et al. 2019) | LiTS (Christ 2021) | DNN | 99% |
| Brain cancer | (Sobhaninia et al. 2019) | CE-MRI (Cheng 2021) | DNN | F1 Score: 78% |
| | (Ari and Hanbay 2018) | DICOM (Kwan et al. 1999) | DNN | 97.18% |

# 4  Scope Versus Challenges in Deep Learning for Healthcare

As presented in this chapter, there is an impressive amount of research work apportioned to the study of Deep Learning in healthcare. However, it is quite surprising that real world deployment of these deep learning algorithms is far from ubiquitous (Kelly et al. 2019). Many factors are responsible for this. Firstly, most of the studies in deep learning have been performed on historically labeled data. The true utility of AI algorithms will be realized when they are applied on real time data, as performance is likely to deteriorate when dealing with real world data that differ from the training data (Kelly et al. 2019). Secondly, the metrics used to understand the accuracy of a deep learning model do not translate well into the healthcare domain. While algorithms are judged on parameters like area under the curve, sensitivity and specificity, in healthcare the yardstick is whether the use of the model results in a beneficial change in patient care (Shah and Milstein 2019). Another challenge that may have unforeseen impact is the susceptibility of deep learning models to adversarial attack or manipulation. This attack occurs when an otherwise effective model is manipulated by doped inputs purposefully designed to deceive them. For example, in one study, the models were fooled into labeling images of benign moles as harmful by injecting adversarial noise and through simple rotations (Finlayson et al. 2019) .

Another major roadblock in the way of the widespread acceptance of deep learning methods in healthcare is the sensitivity of data that needs to be shared across internet boundaries for deep learning models to be trained on. The entire methodology of AI systems involves analyzing and comparing specific patient data with large number of data from other patients. Although this data is anonymized and aggregated, there is a requirement for management of consent and legal ownership in collecting and using personal data. This stringency on data protection has been made evident by the European General Data Protection Regulation (GDPR) that was conceived in 2016 and came into force in May 2018 (Regulation 2016).

Below is a study on the scope of deep learning in healthcare along with the challenges faced by the same (Table 2).

**Table 2** Scope vs Challenges in DL for healthcare

| Field | Scope | Challenges |
| --- | --- | --- |
| Cancer detection | With the advent of sophisticated DL algorithms, processing mammogram images through AI is a regular exercise. In many cases they have yielded results at par with human radiologists | Very often, the Deep Neural Networks fail to consider the other physiological aspects of a patient that would be otherwise available to a human physician and hence results lack in accuracy |
| Actionable medical insights | With increasing patient data being generated, there is a lot of scope in churning the patient details and diagnostic data to come up with strong statistical models that can predict very accurately about the health parameters of an individual | With increasing number of devices and lack of unification among the different data carriers, there is a lot of gap in communication between different devices. It is difficult to incorporate a myriad sensors and embedded systems each different from the other, which makes the proceedings expensive |
| Robotics process automation | Surgical robots improve the ability of the surgeons to see and navigate. They create precise and minimally invasive incisions, stitch wounds with accuracy and minimal pain, and so much more. Use of such robots has been legally approved in USA since 2000. They have been growing in numbers and scope and are used in all kinds of procedures such as orthopedics, urology, gynecology, neurology, thoracic, otolaryngology, bariatric, rectal and colon, and even multiple oncology | The current robotic systems are bulky and not versatile enough. There is a need to embrace this technology wisely, contribute to its development and remain critical. Randomized studies comparing open and robotic surgery needs to be conducted to get a good understanding about the success of these systems. (El-Hakim) |
| Drug discovery | AI and ML techniques are increasingly given preference to solve the difficult task of drug development and synthesis. These techniques are very effective at hunting for new pharmaceutical opportunities in the industry. The availability and adaptability of DL models can accelerate future developments via learned features and theory-informed models | There is a dependency on using experimental data for training and validation. Also, because of the presence of a large number of free parameters, these training models represent a complex optimization problem on top of drug synthesis (Lavecchia 2019) |

(continued)

**Table 2** (continued)

| Field | Scope | Challenges |
|-------|-------|-----------|
| Precision medicine | Deep neural networks, AI-driven search algorithms and probabilistic graph models will play a pivotal role in finding precise treatment option for an individual based on his or her personal medical history, lifestyle choices, genetic database, and dynamically changing pathological tests | DL-based precision medicine combines medicine, biology, statistics, and computing. A sustained collaboration across different disciplines and institutions is required to enable research in this domain. Also, there is still skepticism regarding the clinical adoption of DL technologies emanating from the lack of causality and their 'black-box' nature. The inability to understand why an algorithm achieves generalization and performs so well, may be a critical factor inhibiting the clinical translation of DL technologies |

## 5 Conclusion

One of the major roadblocks for widespread adoption of deep learning in health care is their lack of causality and 'black-box' nature (Georgios and Manolis 2019). However, despite the challenges mentioned, researchers are hopeful that AI and specially Deep Learning, will have a positive impact on the different aspects of medicine. AI systems can decrease random variations in clinical practice, improve efficiency and dodge avoidable medical errors that would otherwise affect almost every patient at least once in their lifetime (McGlynn et al. 2015). Deep Learning and AI could help primary care physicians by enabling them to confidently manage a bigger array of complex diseases. Fast and efficient deep learning tools would assist the specialists with superhuman diagnostic performance and disease management. Also, AI can extract new insights from existing data that clinicians are unable to perceive. Examples include the identification of new predictive features for breast cancer prognosis using stromal cells (rather than the cancer cells themselves) (Beck et al. 2011).

This chapter has been written with the hope of familiarizing the readers with the intelligent systems and algorithms that support decision making in healthcare. Through this medium, the decisions and recommendations of a program can be explained to the users and reviewers. This chapter also discusses the scope of duplicating expertise of human specialists and evaluating the same through a direct comparison between the output of the machine and that of the human experts. Needless to say, there will be cases where an experienced human radiologist has to weigh in his or her opinion, but a majority of the work can be automated, thereby decreasing cost, increasing the accessibility of screenings and speed of diagnosis.

# Bibliography

Alakwaa W, Nassef M (2017) Lung cancer detection and classification with 3D convolutional neural network (3D-CNN). Int J Advan Comput Sci Appl

Ardila D, Kiraly AP, Bharadwaj S (2019) End-to-end lung cancer screening with three-dimensional deep learning on low-dose chest computed tomography

Ari A, Hanbay D (2018) Deep learning based brain tumor classification and detection system

Armato S, McLennan G (2015) Data from LIDC-IDRI. Cancer Imaging Arch

Beck A, Sangoi A, Leung S, Marinelli R, Nielsen T (2011) Systematic analysis of breast cancer morphology uncovers stromal features associated with survival

Bengio Y, Courville A, Vinvent P (2013) Representation learning: a review and new perspectives. IEEE

Booz AH (2017) Data science bowl. Available: https://www.kaggle.com/c/data-science-bowl-2017

"CAMELYON16" (2016) Available: https://camelyon16.grand-challenge.org/Home/

Carolina UO (2021) IDA. Retrieved from http://ida.loni.usc.edu/

Cheng J (2017) Brain tumor dataset. Available: https://doi.org/10.6084/m9.figshare.1512427

Christ P (2021) LiTS—liver tumor segmentation challenge (LiTS17). Available: http://academict orrents.com/details/27772adef6f563a1ecc0ae19a528b956e6c803ce

Das A, Acharya U, Panda S, Sabut S (2019) Deep learning based liver cancer detection using watershed transform and Gaussian mixture model techniques

Doi K (2007) Computer-aided diagnosis in medical imaging: historical review, current status and future potential, Elsevier

El-Hakim A (2007) Challenges of robotic surgery. Canadian Urological Association Journal.

Eltoukhy M, Faye I, Samir B (2010) Breast cancer diagnosis in digital mammogram using multiscale curve let transform

Exchange GH (2017) Global burden of disease collaborative network. Retrieved from http://ghdx. healthdata.org/gbd-results-tool

Fauw J, Ledsam JR, Romera-Paredes B, Nikolov S (2018) Clinically applicable deep learning for diagnosis and referral in retinal disease

Finlayson S, Bowers J, Ito J, Zittrain J (2019) Adversarial attacks on medical machine learning

Georgios Z, Manolis T (2019) Deep learning opens new horizons in personalized medicine

Ginneken B, Hahn H, Meine H (2019) Deep learning based automatic liver tumor segmentation in CT with shape-based post-processing

Gruber N, Antholzer S, Jaschke W, Kremser C, Haltmeier M (2019) A joint deep learning approach for automated liver and tumor segmentation

Hosny A (2018) Deep learning for lung cancer prognostication: a retrospective multi-cohort radiomics study. Available: https://journals.plos.org/plosmedicine/article?id=10.1371/journal. pmed.1002711

Hosny A, Chintan P (2018) Artificial intelligence in radiology

Hosny A, Parmar C, Coroller T, Grossmann P, Zeleznik R, Kumar A (2018) Deep learning for lung cancer prognostication: a retrospective multi-cohort radiomics study. In: PLOS medicine

Jalalian A, Mashohor S, Mahmud R, Karasfi B (2017) Foundation and methodologies in computer-aided diagnosis systems for breast cancer detection

Jakimovski G, Davcev D (2019) Using double convolution neural network for lung cancer stage detection. Appl Sci

Kleene (1956) Representation of events in nerve nets and finite automata

Koza J, Bennett F, Andre D (1996) Automated design of both the topology and sizing of analog electrical circuits using genetic programming. Artific Intell Des

Kelly C, Karthikesalingam A, Suleyman M, Corrado G, King D (2019) Key challenges for delivering clinical impact with artificial intelligence. BMC Med

Kwan R, Evanc A, Pike G (1999) MRI simulation-based evaluation of image-processing and classification methods. IEEE Trans Med Imaging. Retrieved from Pubmed

Lavecchia A (2019) Deep learning in drug discovery: opportunities, challenges and future prospects. Drug Discov Today 24(10):2017–2032

Lee S, Celik S, Logsdon B, Lundberg S (2018) A machine learning approach to integrate big data for precision medicine in acute myeloid leukemia. Nat Commun

Le H, Gupta R, Hou L, Abousamra S, Fassler D, Kurc T (2019) Utilizing automated breast cancer detection to identify spatial distributions of tumor infiltrating lymphocytes in invasive breast cancer. Am J Pathol

Le H (2020) Tumor infitrating lynphocytes. Retrieved from github: https://mathbiol.github.io/tcg atil/

Lyman K "Enlitic homepage" (2021) Available: https://www.enlitic.com/

Mammographic Image Analysis Homepage (2021) Available: http://www.mammoimage.org/dat abases/

Microsoft (2020) Project InnerEye—medical imaging AI to empower clinicians. [Online]. Available: https://www.microsoft.com/en-us/research/project/medical-image-analysis/

McGlynn E, McDonald K, Cassel C (2015) Measurement is essential for improving diagnosis and reducing diagnostic error: a report from the institute of medicine

Medgift, Implementing bidirectional relevance scores for digital histopathology (2021) Available: https://github.com/medgift/iMIMIC-RCVs

Mitchell T (1997) Machine learning. McGraw Hill

National Cancer Institute (2021) Available: https://seer.cancer.gov/

NA (2019) A overview, ScienceDirect topics

Nikolov S, Blackwell S, Mendes R, Fauw J (2018) Deep learning to achieve clinically applicable segmentation of head and neck anatomy for radiotherapy

Omar A, Bakr A, Ibrahima N (2020) Female medical students' awareness, attitudes, and knowledge about early detection of breast cancer in Syrian Private University, Syria. Heliyon

Poole D, Mackworth A, Goebel R (1998) Computational intelligence and knowledge

Regulation (EU) (2016) 2016/679 of the European parliament and of the council

Shah N, Milstein A (2019) Making machine learning models clinically useful

Sobhaninia Z, Rezaei S, Noroozi A, Ahmadi M (2019) Brain tumor segmentation using deep learning by type specific sorting of image

Suckling J (2021) The mini-MIAS database of mammograms. Retrieved from http://peipa.essex. ac.uk/info/mias.html

Tariq N (2018) Breast cancer detection using artificial neural networks

Teakde R, Rajeshwari K (2018) Lung cancer detection and classification using deep learning. In: 2018 Fourth international conference on computing communication control and automation (ICCUBEA). Pune, India

UConn Health Sciences Library (2021) Retrieved from UConn: https://lib.uconn.edu/health/find/ databases/

WHO (2021) WHO News Room. Retrieved from https://www.who.int/news-room/fact-sheets/det ail/cancer

Wu N, Phang J, Park J, Shen Y, Huang Z, Zorin M (2019) Deep neural networks improve radiologists' performance in breast cancer screening

Xu Y, Hosny A, Zeleznik R, Parmar C, Coroller T, Franco I (2019) Deep learning predicts lung cancer treatment response from serial medical imaging. In: Clinical cancer research

Zheng Y, Yang C, Merkulov A (2018) Breast cancer screening using convolutional neural network and follow-up digital mammography

# Deep Learning in Biomedical Text Mining: Contributions and Challenges

**Tanvir Alam and Sebastian Schmeier**

**Abstract** A large number of biomedical texts are published every day in scientific literature. Finding the relevant and useful information from the massive collection of scientific literature is a challenging task that can be compared to finding needles in the haystack. Biomedical text mining is one of the sophisticated methodologies that leverage the extraction of knowledge from existing biomedical texts automatically. Deep learning (DL) based techniques have rejuvenated this field with huge prospects. In this chapter, we highlighted the contribution of DL based techniques in three specific tasks in the field of biomedical text mining: named-entity recognition, relationship extraction, and question answering. We also discussed the DL based models that are proven to be successful in multiple natural language processing tasks and the related challenges we face using such DL based techniques. We believe DL based methods will play a significant role in the coming years for biomedical text mining.

**Keywords** Deep learning · Natural Language Processing · Named-entity recognition · Relationship extraction · Question answering

## 1 Introduction

Biomedical texts and literature are the key knowledge distribution channels for novel scientific findings. More than 3000 new articles are being published every day (Lee et al. 2019) leading to an overwhelming amount of new information for researchers in the biomedical domain (Giorgi and Bader 2018). Extracting relevant scientific information and discovering connections among biomedical entities is a daunting manual task (Jensen et al. 2006). Consequently, automated literature mining, including natural language processing (NLP), has become an integral part

T. Alam (✉)
College of Science and Engineering, Hamad Bin Khalifa University, Doha, Qatar
e-mail: talam@hbku.edu.qa

S. Schmeier
School of Natural and Computational Sciences, Massey University, Auckland, New Zealand

© Springer Nature Switzerland AG 2021
M. Househ et al. (eds.), *Multiple Perspectives on Artificial Intelligence in Healthcare*,
Lecture Notes in Bioengineering, https://doi.org/10.1007/978-3-030-67303-1_14

of biomedical discovery that aids in rapidly accessing novel knowledge contained in large volumes of scientific literature. There are many different tasks related to biomedical text mining, but the most fundamental and useful tasks are named-entity recognition (NER), relation extraction (RE) and question answering (QA) (Lee et al. 2019). Historically, different rule-based (Ananiadou 1994; Dagan and Church 1994), dictionary-based (Salhi et al. 2017) and traditional machine-learning based methods have been used for providing solutions for these tasks. But such methods are heavily dependent on hand-curated features, which are often incomplete and very time-consuming to collect.

Recently, deep learning (DL), a branch of machine learning, has rejuvenated the field of biomedical text mining, including biomedical NLP (BioNLP). The major advantage of DL-based methods over existing methods is that DL-based methods require only a minimal level of hand-curated feature engineering and usually provide much better results, compared to traditional methods. Thus DL, a bio inspired neural network, which deploys multiple layers of artificial neurons to learn hierarchical representation of the data (Chen et al. 2018), is now considered the best paradigm for many different recognition tasks in many scientific domains (Bengio et al. 2013), including BioNLP. More recently, a variety of DL based methods and network architectures have been employed in the context of NLP (Young et al. 2018).

In one of the earliest landmark studies, Collobert et al. showed that DL-based methods can outperform traditional methods in most of the NLP related tasks (Collobert et al. 2011). Since then, DL in NLP has developed a strong following and, additionally, due to the emergence of the concept of word embedding (Mikolov et al. 2013a, b) and advancement of different DL methods (Devlin et al. 2018), it is now being used for all major tasks in NLP and biomedical text processing. In this chapter, we will focus on recent advancements in DL-based methods for biomedical text processing. The structure of this chapter is as follows: Sect. 2 lists DL-based techniques that have commonly been used in biomedical text mining. Sections 3, 4 and 5 discuss the contributions of DL in three key areas of biomedical text processing, namely NER, RE and QA systems. In Sect. 6, we highlight some challenges researchers may face when applying DL based techniques in NLP. Finally, we summarized and concluded the chapter in Sect. 7.

## 2 Deep Learning Architectures and Techniques that Have Been Proven Successful in NLP

In this section, we will first discuss embedding techniques, which are considered the first step in DL-based NLP. Afterwards, we will briefly describe some classical models that have been used for DL-based NLP. Finally, we will briefly describe some state-of-the-art DL techniques that have been published recently and achieved groundbreaking results in NLP.

## 2.1 Embeddings

Embedding is a set of feature engineering and language modeling techniques for NLP where each unit (e.g. word, sentence etc.) of the language are mapped to a vector of numbers. For any language modelling task, it is essential to learn the joint probability distribution of such units from input text (Young et al. 2018). However, such learning suffers from the curse of dimensionality as the data size is huge. As an alternative, distributed representations of input texts have been proposed in low dimensional space (Bengio et al. 2003). Learning the character-, word- or sentence-representations is a crucial step in biomedical text processing. Previous studies focused on learning word representations in a context independent manner. However, recent studies have focused on context-dependent representation learning (e.g. ELMo (Peters et al. 2018), CoVe (McCann et al. 2017)).

Distributional representation of words (word embedding) is often considered the first step in DL-based text processing. Word embedding captures the similarity between words based on the hypothesis that words with a similar meaning tend to appear together in similar context. In DL-based models, words, phrases and sentences are usually represented by embedding. The most successful and popular word embedding, Word2vec, was proposed by Mikolov et al. (2013a, b). The authors proposed a continuous bag of words (CBOW) and skip-gram model to build the distributed representation model. GloVe, proposed by Pennington et al., is another example of word embedding (Pennington et al. 2014). GloVe is essentially a count based model which considers a word co-occurrence matrix as input and this matrix is then factorized to generate a low dimensional representation of words.

Word embedding is a very useful tool to extract syntactic and semantic information from text, but intra-word morphological information might be useful for some specific tasks like NER and parts of speech (POS) tagging (Young et al. 2018). Moreover, in some languages (e.g. Chinese), sentences are not composed of multiple words but individual characters. For such languages character level embedding is a better approach to avoid word segmentation (Chen et al. 2015). For example, Peng et al. have used character-level embedding for sentiment classification (Peng et al. 2017). Additionally out-of-the-vocabulary words can not account for relevant tokens and misspellings (Giorgi and Bader 2018) and character-based embedding is a viable option to tackle such challenges (Ling et al. 2015).

## 2.2 Classical DL Based Techniques: CNN, RNN, LSTM, Attention Mechanism

Convolutional neural networks (CNN) belongs to a class of deep neural networks, which is the most commonly applied technique in DL, owing to its outstanding capacity of capturing spatial information from input data. The basic structure of a CNN consists of convolution layers, non-linear (activation) layers and pooling layers

(Fig. 1) (Lawrence et al. 1997). A convolution layer captures the local connectivity from different parts of the input data by using the same weight vector (weight-sharing policy). Based on this weight-sharing policy and local connectivity, a convolution layer captures intrinsic patterns from the data. The non-linear layer adds non-linear properties from the feature maps generated by the convolution layer. A pooling layer takes the average or maximum value form the non-overlapping region of the feature map.

In addition to spatial dependency in the data, the network also needs to capture temporal and order dependencies from text. Recurrent neural networks (RNN) are designed to exploit temporal relationships form input data. The basic structure of an RNN is shown in Fig. 2.

Though RNNs are designed to capture dependencies from input sequence data, it is generally not a good choice for capturing long range dependencies, as it tends to be biased towards the most recent input from the previous time step (Bengio et al.

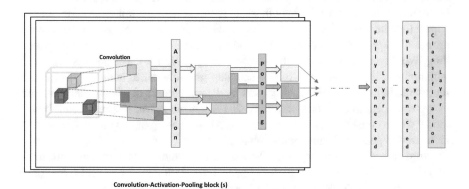

**Fig. 1** A simple convolutional neural network (CNN). The major components of a CNN are: convolutional layers, activation (sigmoid/ReLU) layers, pooling (max/min/average) layers. The surrounding black box around these three layers represents the common order that might be used multiple times to increase the depth of the network. Recent CNNs have more computational layers such as Batch Normalization, Dropout, etc.

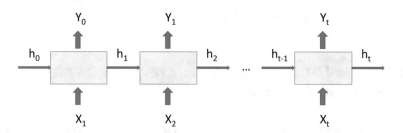

**Fig. 2** A high-level diagram of a recurrent neural network (RNN). Computation at each time step $t$ uses the input $X_t$ and the previous time step's hidden-layer vector $h_{t-1}$ to produce an output $Y_t$ for the current time step and a hidden-layer vector $h_t$ for the next time step

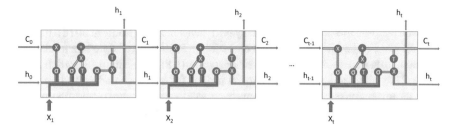

**Fig. 3** An improvement to the vanilla RNN—long short-term memory network. It uses a dedicated memory vector, $C_t$ at each time step to remember certain properties of the input ($X_t$) useful for the task at hand. A combination of the input from the current time-step, the hidden-vector ($h_t$), and the memory from the previous time-step ($C_{t-1}$) are used to compute 'gates' that are used in conjunction with these to produce the hidden-vector and memory values for the next time step

1994). A long short-term memory (LSTM) is a specific RNN, which tries to avoid the pitfalls of an RNN by having memory cells, which store summary information from all the preceding elements of input (Hochreiter and Schmidhuber 1997). A LSTM has a "forget" gate over RNN and this gate allows LSTM to back-propagate the error for unlimited time steps. The basic structure of a LSTM is shown in Fig. 3.

In a traditional sequence-to-sequence model for language translation task, the entire input sentence is encoded into a single vector, which is then used by the decoder to produce the output sentence. This model is not accurate in translating long sentences, since long-term dependencies are difficult to be decoded from a single vector representation of the entire input sentence. To alleviate such problems, attention mechanism has been introduced (Vaswani et al. 2017), where each word in the output sentence depends on a locally weighted combination of the words from the input.

## 2.3 Transfer Learning and Recent DL-Based Architectures that Rejuvenate the NLP Domain

Transfer learning (TL) is the concept to utilize already trained models to perform a similar task on a target dataset (Pan and Yang 2009; Weiss et al. 2016; Day and Khoshgoftaar 2017). TL has been successfully used in many different domains like computer vision (Yosinski et al. 2014; Oquab et al. 2014), speech recognition (Wang and Zheng 2015), etc. Recently, Mou et al. proposed a TL-based method to classify sentences using CNN (Mou et al. 2016). It has been a growing trend in the scientific community of NLP to use embedding with TL (Lee et al. 2019). However for biomedical text mining, the available embedding (e.g. based on wikipedia) needs to be modified to integrate the biomedical vocabulary as there is a huge difference between general corpus text of general corpus (e.g. wikipedia) and a biomedical text corpus (e.g. PubMed, PMC) (Lee et al. 2019).

Generative pre-training (GPT) is a recent model, developed by OpenAI, which achieved state-of-the-art results for many NLP tasks in 2018 (Radford 2018). Instead of using word embedding or character embedding, Radford et al. opted for a subword representation generated by a byte pair encoding (BPE) algorithm (Sennrich et al. 2016). They adopted a semi-supervised approach for language understanding tasks using an unsupervised pre-training approach followed by a supervised fine-tuning approach. In the first stage of model training, a transformer (Vaswani et al. 2017) mechanism was used to learn a universal representation of texts from huge amounts of unlabeled data from a diverse corpus with long stretches of contiguous text. In the second stage of model training, the model was fine tuned using a small amount of labelled data.

Bidirectional encoder representation from transformer (BERT) (Devlin et al. 2018), developed by Google, is a state-of-the-art DL-based word representation model that contextualizes words using bidirectional transfer. BERT proposed that bidirectionally (left-to-right and right-to-left) trained models can have a deeper understanding of the context than single direction language models. BERT uses a masked language model that can predict randomly picked words in a sentence and it showed that the pre-trained representation can reduce the need for a task-specific heavily-engineered DL architecture.

# 3 Deep Learning for Named-Entity Recognition in Biomedical Texts

Named-entity recognition (NER) is the process to recognize and label entities from a given text. NER is one of the most fundamental tasks in biomedical text mining. In the biomedical domain, the most common entity types are genes, proteins, chemicals and diseases (Yoon et al. 2019). NER methods can be broadly categorized into three groups: rule-based, dictionary-based and machine-learning based approaches. Rule based methods are scalable but specific to a particular task and it requires hand curated features and rules to fit into the model (Fukuda et al. 1998; Proux et al. 1998). In the dictionary-based approach, the entity mentioned in the text is checked against a dictionary of words of interest (Salhi et al. 2017; Hettne et al. 2009; Song et al. 2015a). The main drawback of dictionary-based NER is that these methods can not detect out-of-vocabulary words and it is tedious to build an up-to-date dictionary (Yoon et al. 2019). Until recently, NER tools for the biomedical domain were heavily relying on hand curated domain-specific features (Giorgi and Bader 2018). Conditional random fields (CRF) (Lafferty et al. 2001) are considered as the de-facto method for feature-based NER tasks. The process of feature engineering and dictionary creation is time consuming and depends on expert opinions (Leser and Hakenberg 2005) which leads to a domain-specific NER tool which, ultimately, is not generalizable for usage in other domains.

DL-based NER tasks are gaining popularity nowadays due to the advancements of new DL-based architectures that outperform existing rule-based and dictionary-based methods (Crichton et al. 2017; Wang et al. 2019). Recently Habibi et al. proposed a new DL-based long short-term memory network-conditional random field (LSTM-CRF) model which outperformed the state-of-the-art entity specific NER methods (Habibi et al. 2017). Their method combines word embedding, LSTM and CRF into a model for biomedical NER. TL based methods have achieved great attention in the scientific community as they showed significant improvements in NER performance. Lee et al. focused on TL using a CNN for NER (Lee et al. 2017). However, this was not meant for biomedical texts. To the best of our knowledge the first TL-based approach that was applied to biomedical NER was proposed by Giorgi and Bader (2018). Recently, Weber et al. developed HUNER (2019) which is a TL-based method for NER in the biomedical domain. HUNER extended the model proposed by Giorgi and Bader and outperformed the state-of-the-art tools tmChem (Leaman et al. 2015) and GNormPlus (Wei et al. 2015) in recognizing genes, species and chemical entities.

BioBERT, in a recent study gained a lot of attention from the scientific community for NER recognition in biomedical texts (Lee et al. 2019). In BioBERT, Lee et al. considered BERT (Devlin et al. 2018) as the backbone architecture and integrated biomedical articles from Pubmed and PMC with minimal domain-specific architecture modifications to outperform BERT in recognizing four different biomedical entities, genes, drugs, diseases and species.

## 4 Deep Learning for Relationship Extraction from Biomedical Texts

After biomedical entities have been identified in the literature, it is essential to discover underlying relationships among different entities (Rebholz-Schuhmann et al. 2012). Relationship extraction (RE) is meant to determine whether there is an association between entities. This task is more challenging than NER as the RE algorithms need to understand the meaning of a sentence (sentence-level RE) or the meaning within the whole document (document-level RE). RE at document-level is more difficult than sentence-level RE and most of the tools consider sentence-level RE without considering the context from the whole document (Wu et al. 2019).

One of the earliest examples for RE was Diseasome (Goh et al. 2007), where the authors provided the association information regarding 22 categories of human disorders and genes. There are many types of biomedical entities and different solutions have been tailored for identifying association among entities (Rebholz-Schuhmann et al. 2012). The most common type of associations, that is of primary interest for biomedical researchers, are gene-disease associations, protein–protein interactions, drug-drug interactions and gene-variants associations. For such RE tasks, different types of computational methods have been proposed: co-occurrence-based methods

(Hakenberg et al. 2012), pattern-/rule-based methods (Song et al. 2015b), as well as machine-learning based methods (Chun et al. 2006).

The simplest approach to identify a relationship between entities is entity co-occurrence (Stapley and Benoit 2000; Jenssen et al. 2001). A relationship can be inferred if two entities are co-occurring within the same sentence, paragraph, section or a document. Based on co-occurrence, Hakenberg et al. proposed an automated method to create a repository, SNPshot, that highlights genetic variants and their associations to different drugs and diseases (Hakenberg et al. 2012). Salhi et al. developed a knowledgebase, DES-ncRNA, based on 19 topic-specific dictionaries, to find associations between non-coding RNAs (micro-RNAs and long non-coding RNAs) and other entities, including diseases, mutations etc. (Salhi et al. 2017). Rule-based methods have been investigated for a long time for RE tasks from biomedical texts. Xie et al. developed miRCancer, based on 75 rules, to identify miRNAs that are involved in cancer based on text mining from biomedical literature (Xie et al. 2013). They built their own dictionary, regular expressions and rules to capture miRNA expressions and find their association to cancer. Song et al. developed a public knowledge discovery tool, called PKDE4J, to identify entities and extract relationships between entities (Song et al. 2015b). PKDE4J extends the Stanford CoreNLP (Manning et al. 2014) for dictionary-based NER and rule-based RE. Interested readers may refer to the publication (Song et al. 2015b) to understand more details about rule-based RE. Traditional machine-learning-based methods provided many sophisticated solutions for different RE tasks (Leach et al. 2009). Examples of such RE tasks include, but are not limited to, protein–protein interactions (Bui et al. 2011), protein subcellular localization prediction (Brady and Shatkay 2008), gene-disease associations (Chun et al. 2006), drug-drug interactions (Bui et al. 2014), etc.

Recently DL-based methods have gained a lot of attention in RE from biomedical texts. For extracting gene-disease associations from biomedical texts, Wu et al. developed RENET (Wu et al. 2019), a DL-based framework that not only captures sentence-level associations between genes and diseases but also models gene-disease associations across sentences in a document. In RENET, sentence-level representations were computed based on Word2Vec embedding (Mikolov et al. 2013a) and then passed through a CNN. Afterwards the sentence-level representations are transformed into document-level representations through an RNN. Finally, the document-based representation is used for gene-disease association prediction. BioBERT, mentioned above, uses a pre-trained model based on BERT to recognize gene-disease association in biomedical literature (Lee et al. 2019). BioBERT outperformed the state-of-the-art model result for GAD (Bravo et al. 2015) and EU-ADR (Mulligen et al. 2012) datasets in multiple evaluation metrics.

Protein–protein interaction (PPI) extraction from text is a challenging task, where DL-based methods have been used extensively. The majority of the DL-based PPI extraction tasks are performed by either a CNN (Quan et al. 2016; Peng and Lu 2017; Choi 2018) or RNN (Hsieh et al. 2017; Ahmed et al. 2019). Hua and Quan used the shortest dependency path (SDP) and a CNN to extract PPI from biomedical texts (Hua and Quan 2016). Recently, Zhang et al. proposed a residual CNN network for the PPI extraction task and their method achieved the best result in five benchmark data set ( HPRD50, LLL, IEPA, BioInfer, AIMed) for PPI extraction corpora (Zhang et al. 2019).

DL-based methods have made major contributions in extracting drug-drug inter-action (DDI) extraction from literature. Sahu et al. and Huang et al. developed a two-stage LSTM-based model to extract interaction between drugs from literature (Sahu and Anand 2018; Huang et al. 2017). Once a DDI is discovered, the authors categorized their interaction into one of four different groups: advice, effect, mechanism and interaction. Lim used a LSTM based model to extract DDI and their model outperformed other models on DDI Extraction Challenge'13 test data (Lim et al. 2018). Zhao et al. proposed a CNN based model to extract DDI (Zhao et al. 2016). They used a novel syntax embedding approach along with position specific features and POS features to categorize the DDI into five different categories: advice, effect, mechanism, interaction and negative. Liu et al. developed a multilayer bidirectional LSTM with transfer weight matrix (TWM) and a memory network to classify DDI into multiple types (Liu et al. 2019) and their model outperformed the other methods in DDI Extraction 2013 Task (Segura-Bedmar et al. 2014).

## 5  Deep Learning for Question Answering from Biomedical Texts

Question answering (QA) is the process of extracting answers to a specific question given one or multiple contexts (Wiese et al. 2017). The task of QA has been addressed in both, an open domain setup (Voorhees 2001) or domain-specific setup (Tsatsaronis et al. 2015). Based on the experimental setup different datasets have been proposed for the QA task. Stanford Question Answering Dataset (SQuAD) is the largest collection of QA dataset based on Wikipedia articles. SQuAD v1.0 dataset contains ~108 thousand QA pairs (Rajpurkar et al. 2016). However SQuAD is a generic dataset for QA and not specific to the biomedical domain. BioASQ is the most matured QA dataset in the biomedical domain, which comprises ~900 single answers (factoid) or multiple answers (list) question answering (QA) instances (Tsatsaronis et al. 2015).

Traditional QA systems can be divided into multiple modules: NER, question classification, and correct answer processing (Jurafsky and Martin 2009). Such systems have been applied to biomedical QA with limited success. For example Zi et al. developed the OAQA system, which integrates domain-specific information (Yang et al. 2016). Recently, due to the advancement of neural network-based DL techniques, scientific communities are developing end-to-end QA systems, rather than the traditional approach of subdividing the QA system into multiple discrete steps (Wiese et al. 2017). This end-to-end neural QA system usually starts with an embedding layer. Afterwards, an encoding layer is used to process the token vectors, usually by an RNN. The third layer is usually the interaction layer, which captures interactions between questions and contexts. Finally, an answering layer assigns scores for all the context tokens. A list of such neural QA systems is proposed in Wiese et al. (2017), Xiong et al. (2016), Seo et al. (2016), Weissenborn et al. (2017), Wang and Jiang (2016).

Recently, Du et al. proposed a hierarchical attention-based transfer learning model to build a QA system for the biomedical domain (Du et al. 2019). Authors adopted BERT to enrich the semantic representation and a dot-product based attention mechanism to capture the question interaction clues for passage encoding. Their system achieved state-of-the-art performance and outperformed existing solutions for factoid questions (in 2016) and BioASQ-Task B (in 2017). Weissenborn et al. developed FastQA, an RNN-based neural QA system for extractive QA (Weissenborn et al. 2017). In FastQA, authors proposed that to build a high performance QA system, context/type matching heuristics should be considered, as well as more complex composition functions, instead of simple bag of words models. Wiese et al. employed several transfer learning techniques to develop a neural QA system, which achieved state-of-the-art results on factoid QA and good results on a list questions (Wiese et al. 2017). Recently, Lee et al. developed a QA system, which is a part of BioBERT (Lee et al. 2019), by fine tuning the BERT system. For biomedical QA systems, Lee et al. used BioASQ to adopt the same structure of BERT. On all the BioASQ datasets (4b, 5b, 6b), BioBERT outperformed the existing models, considering the mean reciprocal rank (MRR) evaluation metric. Table 1 summarizes DL-based techniques that have been used for NER, RE and QA tasks in biomedical texts and literature.

# 6 Challenges and Future Perspectives

No single method is universally applicable in all NLP domains and the choice of how to use DL techniques is still problem-specific and challenging. Traditional approaches for biomedical text processing will definitely remain valid because of their advantage to succeed even with small amounts of data. Also, to assess the statistics of any finding is still difficult in DL-based techniques (Angermueller et al. 2016). Additionally, the training complexity (e.g. hyperparameter tuning, avoiding overfitting etc.) for DL-based models are much higher compared to traditional machine learning based approaches, which is a common pitfall for all DL techniques. QA tasks from biomedical text are still far away from maturity and likely still a long way off before a mature system emerges. In the last few years, we have observed outstanding conversational agents appearing on the market (e.g., Microsoft Cortana, Apple Siri). But these agents can perform a relatively simple task of answering factual questions (Dhingra et al. 2017). Lack of ability to learn from interactions with a user is the bottleneck in the QA task and reinforcement learning (RL) based techniques will play a big part in the improvement of existing QA systems (Dhingra et al. 2017). In the future, we will expect a lot of improvement and application of DL-based techniques in the QA tasks. Such an improved QA system will play a pivotal role in implementing highly accurate and useful chatbots in the healthcare sector as well. But such systems

**Table 1** Brief list of recent publications and DL-based techniques that have been used in different BioNLP tasks

| Tasks related to BioNLP | Deep learning based techniques | References |
| --- | --- | --- |
| NER | Deep neural network | Yoon et al. (2019) |
| | CNN | Crichton et al. (2017) |
| | RNN/LSTM | Wang et al. (2019), Habibi et al. (2017), Weber et al. (2019) |
| | Transfer learning | Lee et al. (2019), Giorgi and Bader (2018) |
| RE | CNN | Gene-disease (Wu et al. 2019) PPI (Quan et al. 2016; Peng and Lu 2017; Choi 2018; Hua and Quan 2016; Zhang et al. 2019) DDI (Zhao et al. 2016) |
| | RNN/LSTM | PPI (Hsieh et al. 2017; Ahmed et al. 2019) DDI (Sahu and Anand 2018; Huang et al. 2017; Lim et al. 2018; Liu et al. 2019) |
| | Transfer learning | Lee et al. (2019) |
| QA | RNN/LSTM | Wiese et al. (2017), Xiong et al. (2016), Seo et al. (2016), Weissenborn et al. (2017), Wang and Jiang (2016) |
| | Transfer learning | Lee et al. (2019), Wiese et al. (2017), Du et al. (2019) |

need to be significantly enhanced and tested rigorously before applying into real-life clinical setup.

# 7    Conclusions

Deep learning is a useful technique, which has facilitated manifold improvements in biomedical text processing. In this article, we have provided a brief summary of some of the DL-based techniques and their contributions in three key areas of biomedical text processing: NER, RE and QA. This article does not cover all aspects of DL (e.g. deep reinforcement learning) and all tasks related to NLP. However, we focused on the most relevant DL-based techniques that have been used in BioNLP, recently. We believe this article will aid the research community to have an overview of the contributions of DL in biomedical text processing.

**Acknowledgements** We would like to thank Mohammad Tariqul Islam and Faisal Ahmed for the discussion on multiple topics of NLP.

# References

Ahmed M, Islam J, Samee MR, Mercer RE (2019) Identifying Protein-protein interaction using tree LSTM and structured attention. In: 2019 IEEE 13th international conference on semantic computing (ICSC). 2019. https://doi.org/10.1109/icosc.2019.8665584

Ananiadou S (1994) A methodology for automatic term recognition. In: Proceedings of the 15th conference on computational linguistics. https://doi.org/10.3115/991250.991317

Angermueller C, Pärnamaa T, Parts L, Stegle O (2016) Deep learning for computational biology. Mol Syst Biol 12:878

Bengio Y, Simard P, Frasconi P (1994) Learning long-term dependencies with gradient descent is difficult. IEEE Trans Neural Netw 5:157–166

Bengio Y, Ducharme R, Vincent P, Jauvin C (2003) A Neural probabilistic language model. J Mach Learn Res 3:1137–1155

Bengio Y, Courville A, Vincent P (2013) Representation learning: a review and new perspectives. IEEE Trans Pattern Anal Mach Intell 35:1798–1828

Brady S, Shatkay H (2008) EpiLoc: a (working) text-based system for predicting protein subcellular location. Pac Symp Biocomput 604–615

Bravo À, Piñero J, Queralt N, Rautschka M, Furlong LI (2015) Extraction of relations between genes and diseases from text and large-scale data analysis: implications for translational research. https://doi.org/10.1101/007443

Bui Q-C, Katrenko S, Sloot PMA (2011) A hybrid approach to extract protein-protein interactions. Bioinformatics 27:259–265

Bui Q-C, Sloot PMA, van Mulligen EM, Kors JA (2014) A novel feature-based approach to extract drug-drug interactions from biomedical text. Bioinformatics 30:3365–3371

Chen X, Xu L, Liu Z, Sun M, Luan H (2015) Joint learning of character and word embeddings. In: Twenty-fourth international joint conference on artificial intelligence. Available: https://www.aaai.org/ocs/index.php/IJCAI/IJCAI15/paper/view/11000

Chen L-C, Papandreou G, Kokkinos I, Murphy K, Yuille AL (2018) DeepLab: semantic image segmentation with deep convolutional nets, atrous convolution, and fully connected CRFs. IEEE Trans Pattern Anal Mach Intell 40:834–848

Choi S-P (2018) Extraction of protein–protein interactions (PPIs) from the literature by deep convolutional neural networks with various feature embeddings. J Inf Sci 60–73. https://doi.org/10.1177/0165551516673485

Chun H-W, Tsuruoka Y, Kim J-D, Shiba R, Nagata N, Hishiki T et al (2006) Extraction of gene-disease relations from Medline using domain dictionaries and machine learning. Pac Symp Biocomput 4–15

Collobert R, Weston J, Bottou L, Karlen M, Kavukcuoglu K, Kuksa P (2011) Natural language processing (Almost) from scratch. J Mach Learn Res 12:2493–2537

Crichton G, Pyysalo S, Chiu B, Korhonen A (2017) A neural network multi-task learning approach to biomedical named entity recognition. BMC Bioinformatics 18:368

Dagan I, Church K (1994) Termight: Identifying and translating technical terminology. In: Proceedings of the fourth conference on applied natural language processing. https://doi.org/10.3115/974358.974367

Day O, Khoshgoftaar TM (2017) A survey on heterogeneous transfer learning. J Big Data. https://doi.org/10.1186/s40537-017-0089-0

Devlin J, Chang M-W, Lee K, Toutanova K (2018) BERT: Pre-training of deep bidirectional transformers for language understanding. Available: http://arxiv.org/abs/1810.04805

Dhingra B, Li L, Li X, Gao J, Chen Y-N, Ahmed F et al (2017) Towards end-to-end reinforcement learning of dialogue agents for information access. In: Proceedings of the 55th annual meeting of the association for computational linguistics, vol 1. Long Papers. https://doi.org/10.18653/v1/p17-1045

Du Y, Pei B, Zhao X, Ji J (2019) Deep scaled dot-product attention based domain adaptation model for biomedical question answering. Methods. https://doi.org/10.1016/j.ymeth.2019.06.024

Fukuda K, Tamura A, Tsunoda T, Takagi T (1998) Toward information extraction: identifying protein names from biological papers. Pac Symp Biocomput 707–718

Giorgi JM, Bader GD (2018) Transfer learning for biomedical named entity recognition with neural networks. Bioinformatics 34:4087–4094

Goh K-I, Cusick ME, Valle D, Childs B, Vidal M, Barabási A-L (2007) The human disease network. Proc Natl Acad Sci U S A 104:8685–8690

Habibi M, Weber L, Neves M, Wiegandt DL, Leser U (2017) Deep learning with word embeddings improves biomedical named entity recognition. Bioinformatics 33:i37–i48

Hakenberg J, Voronov D, Nguyên VH, Liang S, Anwar S, Lumpkin B et al (2012) A SNPshot of PubMed to associate genetic variants with drugs, diseases, and adverse reactions. J Biomed Inform 45:842–850

Hettne KM, Stierum RH, Schuemie MJ, Hendriksen PJM, Schijvenaars BJA, van Mulligen EM et al (2009) A dictionary to identify small molecules and drugs in free text. Bioinformatics 25:2983–2991

Hochreiter S, Schmidhuber J (1997) Long short-term memory. Neural Comput 1735–1780. https://doi.org/10.1162/neco.1997.9.8.1735

Hsieh Y-L, Chang Y-C, Chang N-W, Hsu W-L (2017) Identifying protein-protein interactions in biomedical literature using recurrent neural networks with long short-term memory. In: Proceedings of the Eighth international joint conference on natural language processing, vol 2. Short Papers, 240–245

Hua L, Quan C (2016) A shortest dependency path based convolutional neural network for protein-protein relation extraction. Biomed Res Int 2016:8479587

Huang D, Jiang Z, Zou L, Li L (2017) Drug–drug interaction extraction from biomedical literature using support vector machine and long short term memory networks. Inf Sci 100–109. https://doi.org/10.1016/j.ins.2017.06.021

Jensen LJ, Saric J, Bork P (2006) Literature mining for the biologist: from information retrieval to biological discovery. Nat Rev Genet 7:119–129

Jenssen T-K, Lægreid A, Komorowski J, Hovig E (2001) A literature network of human genes for high-throughput analysis of gene expression. Nat Genet 21–28. https://doi.org/10.1038/ng0501-21

Jurafsky D, Martin JH (2009) Speech and language processing: an introduction to natural language processing, computational linguistics, and speech recognition. Prentice Hall

Lafferty JD, McCallum A, Pereira FCN (2001) Conditional random fields: probabilistic models for segmenting and labeling sequence data. In: Proceedings of the eighteenth international conference on machine learning. Morgan Kaufmann Publishers Inc., pp 282–289

Lawrence S, Giles CL, Tsoi AC, Back AD (1997) Face recognition: a convolutional neural-network approach. IEEE Trans Neural Netw 98–113. https://doi.org/10.1109/72.554195

Leach SM, Tipney H, Feng W, Baumgartner WA, Kasliwal P, Schuyler RP et al (2009) Biomedical discovery acceleration, with applications to craniofacial development. PLoS Comput Biol. 2009;5: e1000215

Leaman R, Wei C-H, Lu Z (2015) tmChem: a high performance approach for chemical named entity recognition and normalization. J Cheminform 7:S3

Lee JY, Dernoncourt F, Szolovits P (2017) Transfer learning for named-entity recognition with neural networks. Available: http://arxiv.org/abs/1705.06273

Lee J, Yoon W, Kim S, Kim D, Kim S, So CH et al (2019) BioBERT: a pre-trained biomedical language representation model for biomedical text mining. Bioinformatics. https://doi.org/10.1093/bioinformatics/btz682

Leser U, Hakenberg J (2005) What makes a gene name? Named entity recognition in the biomedical literature. Brief Bioinform 6:357–369

Lim S, Lee K, Kang J (2018) Drug drug interaction extraction from the literature using a recursive neural network. PLoS ONE. e0190926. https://doi.org/10.1371/journal.pone.0190926

Ling W, Dyer C, Black AW, Trancoso I, Fermandez R, Amir S et al (2015) Finding function in form: compositional character models for open vocabulary word representation. In: Proceedings

of the 2015 conference on empirical methods in natural language processing. https://doi.org/10.
18653/v1/d15-1176

Liu J, Huang Z, Ren F, Hua L (2019) Drug-drug interaction extraction based on transfer weight
matrix and memory network. IEEE Access 101260–101268. https://doi.org/10.1109/access.2019.
2930641

Manning C, Surdeanu M, Bauer J, Finkel J, Bethard S, McClosky D (2014) The stanford CoreNLP
natural language processing toolkit. In: Proceedings of 52nd annual meeting of the association
for computational linguistics: system demonstrations. https://doi.org/10.3115/v1/p14-5010

McCann B, Bradbury J, Xiong C, Socher R (2017) Learned in translation: contextualized word
vectors. Adv Neural Inf Proc Syst 6294–6305

Mikolov T, Sutskever I, Chen K, Corrado GS, Dean J (2013a) Distributed representations of words
and phrases and their compositionality. Adv Neural Inform Proc Syst 3111–3119

Mikolov T, Chen K, Corrado G, Dean J (2013b) Efficient estimation of word representations in
vector space. Available: http://arxiv.org/abs/1301.3781

Mou L, Meng Z, Yan R, Li G, Xu Y, Zhang L et al (2016) How transferable are neural networks
in NLP Applications? In: Proceedings of the 2016 conference on empirical methods in natural
language processing. https://doi.org/10.18653/v1/d16-1046

Oquab M, Bottou L, Laptev I, Sivic J (2014) Learning and transferring mid-level image representations using convolutional neural networks. In: 2014 IEEE conference on computer vision and
pattern recognition. https://doi.org/10.1109/cvpr.2014.222

Pan SJ, Yang Q (2009) A survey on transfer learning. IEEE J Mag. [cited 28 Sep 2019]. Available:
https://ieeexplore.ieee.org/abstract/document/5288526

Peng Y, Lu Z (2017) Deep learning for extracting protein-protein interactions from biomedical
literature. BioNLP 2017. https://doi.org/10.18653/v1/w17-2304

Peng H, Cambria E, Zou X (2017) Radical-based hierarchical embeddings for Chinese sentiment
analysis at sentence level. In: The Thirtieth international flairs conference. Available: https://
www.aaai.org/ocs/index.php/FLAIRS/FLAIRS17/paper/view/15460

Pennington J, Socher R, Manning C (2014) Glove: global vectors for word representation. In:
Proceedings of the 2014 conference on empirical methods in natural language processing
(EMNLP). https://doi.org/10.3115/v1/d14-1162

Peters M, Neumann M, Iyyer M, Gardner M, Clark C, Lee K et al (2018) Deep contextualized word
representations. In: Proceedings of the 2018 conference of the North American chapter of the
association for computational linguistics: human language technologies, vol 1. (Long Papers).
https://doi.org/10.18653/v1/n18-1202

Proux D, Rechenmann F, Julliard L, Pillet VV, Jacq B (1998) Detecting gene symbols and names
in biological texts: a first step toward pertinent information extraction. Genome Inform Ser
Workshop Genome Inform 9:72–80

Quan C, Hua L, Sun X, Bai W (2016) Multichannel convolutional neural network for biological
relation extraction. Biomed Res Int 2016:1850404

Radford A (2018) Improving language understanding by generative pre-training. [cited 28 Sep
2019]. Available: https://pdfs.semanticscholar.org/cd18/800a0fe0b668a1cc19f2ec95b5003d0a5
035.pdf

Rajpurkar P, Zhang J, Lopyrev K, Liang P (2016) SQuAD: 100,000 questions for machine comprehension of text. In: Proceedings of the 2016 conference on empirical methods in natural language
processing. https://doi.org/10.18653/v1/d16-1264

Rebholz-Schuhmann D, Oellrich A, Hoehndorf R (2012) Text-mining solutions for biomedical
research: enabling integrative biology. Nat Rev Genet 13:829–839

Sahu SK, Anand A (2018) Drug-drug interaction extraction from biomedical texts using long
short-term memory network. J Biomed Inform 86:15–24

Salhi A, Essack M, Alam T, Bajic VP, Ma L, Radovanovic A et al (2017) DES-ncRNA: A knowledgebase for exploring information about human micro and long noncoding RNAs based on
literature-mining. RNA Biol 14:963–971

Segura-Bedmar I, Martínez P, Herrero-Zazo M (2013) Lessons learnt from the DDIExtraction-2013 shared task. J Biomed Inform 152–164. https://doi.org/10.1016/j.jbi.2014.05.007

Sennrich R, Haddow B, Birch A (2016) Neural machine translation of rare words with subword units. In: Proceedings of the 54th annual meeting of the association for computational linguistics, vol 1. Long Papers. https://doi.org/10.18653/v1/p16-1162

Seo M, Kembhavi A, Farhadi A, Hajishirzi H (2016) Bidirectional attention flow for machine comprehension. Available: http://arxiv.org/abs/1611.01603

Song M, Yu H, Han W-S (2015a) Developing a hybrid dictionary-based bio-entity recognition technique. BMC Med Inform Decis Mak 15(Suppl 1):S9

Song M, Kim WC, Lee D, Heo GE, Kang KY (2015b) PKDE4J: entity and relation extraction for public knowledge discovery. J Biomed Inform 57:320–332

Stapley BJ, Benoit G (2000) Biobibliometrics: information retrieval and visualization from co-occurrences of gene names in Medline abstracts. Pac Symp Biocomput 529–540

Tsatsaronis G, Balikas G, Malakasiotis P, Partalas I, Zschunke M, Alvers MR et al (2015) An overview of the BIOASQ large-scale biomedical semantic indexing and question answering competition. BMC Bioinf 16:138

van Mulligen EM, Fourrier-Reglat A, Gurwitz D, Molokhia M, Nieto A, Trifiro G et al (2012) The EU-ADR corpus: Annotated drugs, diseases, targets, and their relationships. J Biomed Inf 879–884. https://doi.org/10.1016/j.jbi.2012.04.004

Vaswani A, Shazeer N, Parmar N, Uszkoreit J, Jones L, Gomez AN et al (2017) Attention is all you need. Adv Neural Inf Process Syst 5998–6008

Voorhees EM (2001) The TREC question answering track. Nat Lang Eng, 361–378. https://doi.org/10.1017/s1351324901002789

Wang S, Jiang J (2016) Machine comprehension using match-LSTM and answer pointer. Available: http://arxiv.org/abs/1608.07905

Wang D, Zheng TF (2015) Transfer learning for speech and language processing. In: 2015 Asia-Pacific signal and information processing association annual summit and conference (APSIPA). https://doi.org/10.1109/apsipa.2015.7415532

Wang X, Zhang Y, Ren X, Zhang Y, Zitnik M, Shang J et al (2019) Cross-type biomedical named entity recognition with deep multi-task learning. Bioinformatics 35:1745–1752

Weber L, Münchmeyer J, Rocktäschel T, Habibi M, Leser U (2019) HUNER: improving biomedical NER with pretraining. Bioinformatics. https://doi.org/10.1093/bioinformatics/btz528

Wei C-H, Kao H-Y, Lu Z (2015) GNormPlus: an integrative approach for tagging genes, gene families, and protein domains. Biomed Res Int 2015:918710

Weiss K, Khoshgoftaar TM, Wang D (2016) A survey of transfer learning. J Big Data. https://doi.org/10.1186/s40537-016-0043-6

Weissenborn D, Wiese G, Seiffe L (2017) Making neural QA as simple as possible but not simpler. In: Proceedings of the 21st conference on computational natural language learning (CoNLL 2017). https://doi.org/10.18653/v1/k17-1028

Wiese G, Weissenborn D, Neves M (2017) Neural domain adaptation for biomedical question answering. In: Proceedings of the 21st conference on computational natural language learning (CoNLL 2017). https://doi.org/10.18653/v1/k17-1029

Wu Y, Luo R, Leung HCM, Ting H-F, Lam T-W (2019) RENET: a deep learning approach for extracting gene-disease associations from literature. Lect Notes Comput Sci 272–284. https://doi.org/10.1007/978-3-030-17083-7_17

Xie B, Ding Q, Han H, Wu D (2013) miRCancer: a microRNA-cancer association database constructed by text mining on literature. Bioinformatics 29:638–644

Xiong C, Zhong V, Socher R (2016) Dynamic coattention networks for question answering. Available: http://arxiv.org/abs/1611.01604

Yang Z, Zhou Y, Nyberg E (2016) Learning to answer biomedical questions: OAQA at BioASQ 4B. Proc Fourth BioASQ Workshop. https://doi.org/10.18653/v1/w16-3104

Yoon W, So CH, Lee J, Kang J (2019) CollaboNet: collaboration of deep neural networks for biomedical named entity recognition. BMC Bioinf 20:249

Yosinski J, Clune J, Bengio Y, Lipson H (2014) How transferable are features in deep neural networks? Adv Neural Inf Process Syst 3320–3328

Young T, Hazarika D, Poria S, Cambria E (2018) Recent trends in deep learning based natural language processing [Review Article]. IEEE Comput Intell Mag 55–75. https://doi.org/10.1109/mci.2018.2840738

Zhang H, Guan R, Zhou F, Liang Y, Zhan Z-H, Huang L et al (2019) Deep residual convolutional neural network for protein-protein interaction extraction. IEEE Access. 89354–89365. https://doi.org/10.1109/access.2019.2927253

Zhao Z, Yang Z, Luo L, Lin H, Wang J (2016) Drug drug interaction extraction from biomedical literature using syntax convolutional neural network. Bioinformatics. p. btw486. https://doi.org/10.1093/bioinformatics/btw486

# Artificial Intelligence in the Fight Against the COVID-19 Pandemic: Opportunities and Challenges

**Alaa Abd-Alrazaq, Jens Schneider, Dari Alhuwail, Mounir Hamdi, Saif Al-Kuwari, Dena Al-Thani, and Mowafa Househ**

**Abstract** The world is witnessing unprecedented times as the novel Coronavirus disease (COVID-19) has already conquered and locked down most of the globe. While some indications suggest that the COVID-19 curve is starting to flatten, as of May 2020, we still see constant linear growth in cases and fatalities. Even worse, it is speculated that the situation may further deteriorate with a possible second wave. As governments around the world continue to impose increasingly stringent measures to fight and limit the spread of the pandemic, Artificial Intelligence (AI) tools can play a significant role in the public health surveillance and diagnostics relating to COVID-19. AI is being heavily leveraged in the diagnosis of COVID-19, prediction of its severity for infection, and the discovery of related drugs and vaccines. However, several challenges can impede the exploitation of AI amid the COVID-19 pandemic such as lack of data, privacy, and maturity of AI applications.

A. Abd-Alrazaq · J. Schneider · M. Hamdi · S. Al-Kuwari · D. Al-Thani · M. Househ (✉)
Division of Information and Computing Technology, College of Science and Engineering, Hamad Bin Khalifa University, Qatar Foundation, Doha, Qatar
e-mail: mhouseh@hbku.edu.qa

A. Abd-Alrazaq
e-mail: aabdalrazaq@hbku.edu.qa

J. Schneider
e-mail: jeschneider@hbku.edu.qa

M. Hamdi
e-mail: mhamdi@hbku.edu.qa

S. Al-Kuwari
e-mail: smalkuwari@hbku.edu.qa

D. Al-Thani
e-mail: dalthani@hbku.edu.qa

D. Alhuwail
College of Life Sciences, Kuwait University, Kuwait, Kuwait

Health Informatics Unit, Dasman Diabetes Institute, Kuwait, Kuwait

D. Alhuwail
e-mail: dari.alhuwail@ku.edu.kw

© Springer Nature Switzerland AG 2021
M. Househ et al. (eds.), *Multiple Perspectives on Artificial Intelligence in Healthcare*,
Lecture Notes in Bioengineering, https://doi.org/10.1007/978-3-030-67303-1_15

This chapter discusses the main AI opportunities and challenges in the fight against the COVID-19 pandemic.

# 1 Introduction

Caused by the Severe Acute Respiratory Syndrome Coronavirus 2 (SARS-CoV-2), the highly infectious Coronavirus disease (COVID-19) pandemic has been wreaking havoc across the globe with unprecedented high volumes of infections and deaths (World Health Organization 2019). Individuals infected with COVID-19 often experience fever, dry cough, and fatigue; some battle with severe symptoms often requiring intensive care, while others require mechanical ventilation (Rio and Malani 2020). Quickly after COVID-19 broke out in Wuhan, Hubei Province, China in late December 2019 (Kong et al. 2020), the pandemic has created major disruptions to businesses, education, transportation, and nearly every aspect of our daily lives at local, regional, and international levels (Fontanarosa and Bauchner 2020). In March 2020, the World Health Organization (WHO) declared COVID-19 a global pandemic and a major public health emergency (Chen and Li 2020). Public health emergencies, such as COVID-19, necessitate prompt and effective countermeasures to fight the pandemic and flatten its curve; comprehensive public health strategies that involve surveillance, diagnostics, clinical treatments, and vaccine research are required as early as possible (Yang and Wang 2020). There is an urgent call for action by several governments and healthcare systems reaching out to the research community to develop Artificial Intelligence (AI) applications to assist with COVID-19-related endeavors (Alimadadi et al. 2020).

We live in a hyperconnected world in which data is the fuel of the twenty-first century and AI is its refinery. In recent years, AI has been advancing at an exponential rate. AI refers to a branch of computer science concerned with analyzing and handling complex information from various disparate sources in a wide range of applications in various industries (Contreras and Vehi 2018; Shi et al. 2020). For example, AI is able to efficiently and swiftly analyze high-resolution images from drones and satellites to improve emergency response to a humanitarian crisis (Fan et al. 2019). In healthcare, AI methods perform exceptionally well at recognizing complex patterns in imaging data and providing doctors with rich assessments of radiographic characteristics to aid their diagnosis (Hosny et al. 2018). The term AI is often used with other terms such as Machine Learning (ML) and Deep Learning (DL). ML is a subset of AI that leverages statistical methods to learn patterns and relationships from data by using efficient computing algorithms (Deo 2015). DL, on the other hand, which is a subset of ML, is a form of "representation learning", where machines are fed with raw data to develop representations needed for pattern recognition" (Esteva et al. 2019).

While defining the taxonomy of AI is not trivial, its methods can be generally categorized based on the objective sought, as follows: (i) learning from knowledge, (ii) exploring and discovering knowledge, (iii) extracting conclusions and reasoning from knowledge (Contreras and Vehi 2018). Regardless of the type or subset, through the use of algorithms, AI enables machines to become intelligent, understand queries, sift through and connect mountains of data points, and draw actionable conclusions (Russell and Norvig 2010). Despite the hype for leveraging AI for many applications since the 1950s, it is only recently that we witness its power due to the availability and ever increasing high-throughput computing resources as well as the oceans of data generated every second (van Hartskamp et al. 2019). Considering a hierarchical perspective, AI methods can support COVID-19 at different levels: (a) molecular-level (e.g. drug and vaccine discovery); (b) patient-level (e.g. medical treatment and diagnosis); and (c) population-level (e.g. epidemiological prediction and surveillance) (Bullock et al. 2020). However, several challenges can impede the exploitation of AI amid the COVID-19 pandemic such as lack of data, privacy, and maturity of AI applications. This chapter elucidates the main AI opportunities and challenges in the fight against the COVID-19 pandemic.

## 2 AI Potentials in the Fight Against COVID-19

### 2.1 Early Warnings

AI can play an important role in predicting infectious disease outbreaks, thereby, sending early warnings and alerts to countries and individuals. For example, HealthMap and BlueDot are two AI-based tools that analyze many data sources (e.g., official proclamations, online news, eyewitness reports, forums, blogs, and mass media) in different languages to disseminate early warnings about emerging diseases (HealthMap. About HealthMap 2020; Naudé 2020a; Niiler 2020). Both tools outperformed humans in predicting the COVID-19 outbreak. Specifically, HealthMap and BlueDot sounded alerts about the outbreak of a SARS-like disease 9 and 8 days before the World Health Organization, respectively (Naudé 2020a; Bryson 2020). BlueDot also correctly identified 10 of 12 cities that will be at the forefront of the worldwide outbreak of COVID-19 based on travel data from Wuhan Tianhe International Airport (Bryson 2020; Bogoch et al. 2020).

### 2.2 Forecasting the Epidemic Development

Forecasting and tracking the epidemic development of a disease is very important for public health authorities to track their status on the epidemiological curve and the effectiveness of the containment interventions and measures delivered to decrease the spread of the disease (e.g., social distance, curfews, and lockdowns). In such situations, AI can be harnessed in forecasting how the epidemic develops, such as numbers of confirmed, recovered, death, suspected, asymptomatic and critical cases, and length and ending time of the disease. Forecasting the epidemic development can help in applying targeted lockdowns instead of uniform lockdowns, and this, in turn, saves lives of the most vulnerable group, enables less strict lockdowns for the least vulnerable group, and reduces economic losses. Until the 12th of April 2020, there were 14 studies that used AI for forecasting the development of the COVID-19 pandemic (Abd-alrazaq et al. 2020a). Further, numerous dashboards have been developed to visualize the pandemic development such as UpCode dashboard, New York Times dashboard, and NextStrain dashboard (Patel 2020).

## 2.3   Early Detection and Diagnosis

In epidemiology, it is crucial to diagnose a disease as accurate and as fast as possible to limit its spread and save lives. The Reverse Transcription-Polymerase Chain Reaction (RT-PCR) test is widely used for diagnosing COVID-19 (Ai et al. 2019). Yet, the RT-PCR test, especially real-time RT-PCR, produces high rates of false-negative results and requires between 1 and 6 h to show results (based on testing kits developed by different companies) (Ai et al. 2019; Long et al. 2020; Tahamtan and Ardebili 2020). To improve the performance of the RT-PCR test in terms of speed and sensitivity, AI can be integrated with the test to distinguish SARS-CoV-2 from other Coronaviruses based on viral genome sequences (Lopez-Rincon et al. 2020). AI is used to rapidly develop assays that are accurate and cover numerous genomes (Bullock et al. 2020). AI has the potential to accurately and rapidly diagnose COVID-19 cases based on medical imaging such as X-ray and Computed Tomography (CT) (Abd-alrazaq et al. 2020a). Further, public health authorities can use AI for early detection of suspected COVID-19 cases through analyzing various indicators such as respiratory patterns (Wang et al. 2020a), routine laboratory tests (Feng et al. 2020; Meng et al. 2020), body temperature (Naudé 2020b), and clinical signs and symptoms (OECD 2020).

## 2.4   Prognosis Prediction

Once an individual is diagnosed with a disease, it is important to predict its prognosis to identify the treatment plan and allocate the appropriate medical resources. In this regard, AI has the potential to identify the severity of COVID-19 (through quantification of infected regions in lungs shown in X-ray and CT images) and to predict cases that are at high risk of progression to severe COVID-19 (Abd-alrazaq et al. 2020a). Additionally, AI is capable to forecast the mortality risk among COVID-19 cases and the length of their hospital stay (Abd-alrazaq et al. 2020a).

## 2.5    Treatments and Vaccine Development

AI can contribute to and accelerate drug development through predicting protein structures of SARS-COV-2 (e.g., 3C-like protease, helicase, and spike glycoprotein), which can assist in discovering inhibitors for these proteins (Abd-alrazaq et al. 2020a; Naudé 2020b). AI can also be used for repurposing commercially available drugs to combat COVID-19 through constructing biomedical knowledge graphs, which identify the associations between various entities (e.g., drugs, human proteins, and viral proteins) (Bullock et al. 2020). Researchers and scientists can depend on AI to develop a vaccine for COVID-19 (Abd-alrazaq et al. 2020a). AI can be employed to predict the safety of a treatment for COVID-19 (Wang et al. 2020b).

## 2.6    Social Control

To minimize the spread of infectious diseases, societies must follow rules imposed by public health authorities. AI plays a pivotal role in implementing social control amid the COVID-19 pandemic. For instance, AI-based mobile apps, wearables, and computer vision camera systems can be used to ensure that COVID-19 cases comply with self-quarantine commands and to warn those who breach the quarantine. Public health authorities can use computer vision camera systems in public areas to monitor people commitment to social distancing and mask wearing. Using geolocation data, AI-powered mobile apps can work as contact tracing systems to identify individuals who have contacted known COVID-19 cases and to request them to quarantine themselves instantly. Such apps can also identify potential hotspots of the pandemic in real-time and warn individuals approaching them.

## 2.7    Infodemiology

During the COVID-19 pandemic, misinformation and disinformation have widely spread on the Internet and social media platforms (Abd-Alrazaq et al. 2020b). Such information and fake news can ruin public health measures, activities, and plans to combat the pandemic and create mass-panic in societies. AI has an opportunity to reduce misinformation and disinformation posted on the internet. For example, several social media platforms (e.g., Facebook) and search engines (e.g., Google) are harnessing AI to find and remove fake news from their platforms. AI-based mobile apps have been developed to raise awareness of sanitation and hygiene by combining authentic sources (e.g., WHO guidelines) of information with daily news (Pandey et al. 2020).

## 2.8  Other opportunities

AI-powered robots have the potential to reduce the workload and exposure risk of healthcare workers while interacting with COVID-19 cases by cleaning and disinfecting patients' rooms and healthcare facilities, as well as delivering meals, medications, and equipment to them (Bullock et al. 2020; OECD 2020). AI-based chatbots can be used to provide psychological support to COVID-19 patients and individuals in quarantine and their homes (Abd-alrazaq et al. 2019, 2020cs). AI can assist in predicting potential hosts or reservoirs of SARS-COV-2 by analyzing genome sequences of all viruses and their host information (Guo et al. 2019; Randhawa et al. 2020).

# 3  Challenges in Leveraging AI in the Fight Against COVID-19

## 3.1  Data Challenges

Many COVID-19 related surveys have explored the use of AI against COVID-19, and one study, concluded that: "AI has not yet been impactful against COVID-19. Its use is hampered by a lack of data, and by too much data."(Naudé 2020b). While this quote seems paradoxical at first glance, it reflects the reality of AI-based technology use in the fight against COVID-19. On the one hand, as of June 2020, WHO has confirmed almost 6.4 million cases with over 383,000 deaths (World Health Organization 2019). On the other hand, large and complete data sets that would allow for training AI models to a degree of accuracy that would make them useful are still amiss. For instance, MosMed made 1110 chest CT scans publicly available, with 75% COVID-19 positive cases classified by severity (Center of Diagnostics and Telemedicine 2020). The total volume of data amounts to 11.5 gigabytes. And while providing this data to the international research community is laudable, it is also noteworthy that, to reduce data size, nine out of ten CT slices have been removed, and that MosMed hosted a webinar using a much larger data set (Morozov 2020). The dilemma is, simply put, that even woefully incomplete data can be quite large, taking hours to download and even updating a pre-existing deep classification network ("transfer learning") is time consuming.

## 3.2  Maturity and Acceptance Challenges

Worse yet, according to private communications with radiologists, the recent trend of training AIs to predict COVID-19 related pneumonia from other forms of pneumonia is of little value in a clinical setting. The reason is that radiologists can discriminate viral from bacterial pneumonia with high reliability and in little time. The differentiation between COVID-19 related and other forms of viral pneumonia can be achieved in as little as 15 min with serological tests that require very little prior training (Qatar Biomedical Research Institute 2020). However, a combination with other AI-based predictions such as probability for complications or the overall severity of the infection could increase the value of such classifiers dramatically, in particular considering cost and risk of infection when using chest CT scans. Our assessment also resonates with Bullock et al.'s central insight:

> To date, few of the research projects and systems presented are as yet sufficiently mature to be operationalized at scale, with different applications having different timescales of development, validation, and deployment. As a result, it is important for the founders, users, and AI community to map which technologies could assist with the short-term response, mid-term recovery efforts, and the longer-term preparedness for future pandemics. (Naudé 2020b).

It is also striking that the most successful models to predict the spread of COVID-19 or to assess the impact of non-pharmaceutical interventions (NPIs) such as social distancing are not based on AI, but on state transition models such as SIR or SEIR (Susceptible, [Exposed], Infected, Removed) and extensions thereof (Keeling and Rohani 2008). The reason is, simply put, that such models have been under research for more than a decade and are much more accurate and explainable than their more recent AI contenders (Naudé 2020b).

Given the current, quickly-paced research climate in which scientists world-wide seek solutions to successfully end the pandemic, it is thus hardly surprising that large consortiums with the goal of developing autonomous diagnostic AIs are formed (Imaging COVID-19 AI 2020). The reason why we believe such efforts to be valuable is because they propose value past the current pandemic. Even though it seems likely that most of the AI currently being developed will arrive too late to be of use in the current pandemic, technology that encourages or facilitates NPIs will be of long-lasting value in alleviating the effects of seasonal influenza or combating pandemics to come. For instance, the autonomous diagnostic AIs being developed in the current fight against COVID-19 could lead to self-diagnosis protocols in the future, providing medical personnel with new ways to enjoy a safe distance from patients. While autonomous temperature screening and robotic drug delivery already exist, robots administering medical treatment to increase clinical throughput could follow, but require more time to mature. Strikingly, most recent surveys scoping the landscape of AI vs COVID-19 come to the conclusion that many studies are preliminary and results are reported inadequately, up to the point where the experiments in such studies are hardly reproducible (Bullock et al. 2020; Wynants et al. 2020).

## 3.3  Ethical Challenges

As we advance the route of such technological development, ethical and legal questions arise that we need to assess as a society. For instance, is AI a mere tool akin to an x-ray machine or more? Who is liable when using AI? When is it ethically acceptable to replace human knowledge with an AI and which data may be used with or without the patient's consent? And, finally, is it acceptable to trust an AI when we do not yet fully understand its inner workings? The European Commission has taken the first steps in formulating regulations and guidelines regarding these questions (European Commission 2020a, 2020b), but we need more, properly conducted studies on the use of AI in a clinical environment before some of these questions can be answered reliably.

## *3.4  Privacy Challenges*

As AI is increasingly becoming useful in the fight against the COVID-19 pandemic, it is being adopted to many applications, from disease diagnosis and prediction to spread containment. However, not surprisingly, these AI applications raise privacy concerns as they usually require access to personal data, whose importance for the accuracy of the AI is paramount.

While the traditional AI applications dealing with patients have major privacy concerns, the true privacy challenge AI needs to address is manifested by those applications extracting private information from a larger population; contact tracing is a prime example of this class of applications. Clearly, effective contact tracing requires constant access to personal data, such as location traces and other identification information which will inevitably result in privacy implications (Fontanarosa and Bauchner 2020). Unfortunately, for such a process to be effective, most of the population should be actively participating. This drove some governments to introduce new schemes to mandate it, which raised even more privacy concerns.

The urgency of the situation did not allow sufficient time to conduct proper privacy impact assessments, which accordingly forced governments to abruptly take such measures. Nonetheless, it is still extremely important that full transparency is practiced with all individuals affected. Such individuals must be kept fully informed about how and when their data are being used, especially as it seems that we will have to keep fighting this pandemic for months to come. It is also equally important that governments do not take advantage of this situation to use the data for purposes other than related to the pandemic or to keep following more relaxed privacy guidelines even after the pandemic is over. Such practice can lead to serious consequences, where citizens lose trust in their governments, potentially affecting their commitments to government-issued health guidelines and recommendations; and that will, in turn, lead to a degraded public health condition (Naudé 2020b).

## 3.5 Explainable AI

While AI applications seem to have great potential to help in the fight against COVID-19, making the AI system results accessible to the healthcare professionals and decision-makers remains an open problem. Having to trust the outcomes of an AI application is a debatable issue in research (Varshney 2019). In the past few years, there has been increased attention toward the usefulness and fairness of AI-based models (Abdul et al. 2018; Ribeiro et al. 2016). This everlasting societal demand to provide bases of trust and usefulness in AI results (Selbst and Powles 2017) lead the field of Explainable AI (XAI) to emerge. XAI is a new area of research focusing on making the results of AI techniques easy to comprehend, to reproduce, and to improve its trustworthiness by human users. This field brings together perspectives from several different areas, including psychology, cognitive science, and human–computer interaction (Liao et al. 2020). These demands have already resulted in regulation being imposed (Goodman and Flaxman 2017; Wachter et al. 2017). On the global level, efforts have been made, by the International Telecommunication Union and WHO, to form a collaborative working group on AI-Health in an attempt to establish standards and guidelines for wider acceptability and applicability (International Telecommunication Union 2018). Despite the efforts in both research and policy-making spheres, XAI is in its infancy. This has undoubtedly created a challenge in putting these AI systems in use during the fight against the COVID-19 pandemic (VanBerlo and Ross 2020). As this chapter described, there are several promising solutions. Yet, the use of such solutions in real-life scenarios remains subject to the health professional and decision-makers' acceptance and trust.

## 4 Conclusion

AI technologies appear to have great potential to help in the fight against COVID-19. However, several challenges can impede the exploitation of AI amid the COVID-19 pandemic, such as lack of data, immaturity of AI applications, privacy issues, ethical considerations, and lack of trust in AI outcomes. Thus, it seems that most of the AI applications currently being developed will arrive too late to be of use in the current pandemic, but they can be useful in response to a possible second wave of COVID-19 or upcoming pandemics. To speed up the development of AI applications, there is an imperative for sharing medical and biological datasets, AI models/algorithms, and scientific research on open access platforms. Further, developers of AI applications should ensure robustness, trustworthiness, security, and explainability. Lastly, authorities must respect data privacy and individuals' rights by not using the data for purposes other than the pandemic and practicing more relaxed privacy guidelines even after the pandemic is over.

# References

Abd-alrazaq AA, Alajlani M, Alalwan AA, Bewick BM, Gardner P, Househ M (2019) An overview of the features of chatbots in mental health: A scoping review. Int J Med Inf 132:103978, 01 Dec 2019. https://doi.org/10.1016/j.ijmedinf.2019.103978

Abd-alrazaq AA, Alajlani M, Alhuwail D, Schneider J, Al-Kuwari S, Shah Z et al (2020a) Artificial intelligence in the fight against COVID-19: scoping review. J Med Internet Res

Abd-Alrazaq A, Alhuwail D, Househ M, Hamdi M, Shah Z (2020b) Top concerns of tweeters during the COVID-19 pandemic: infoveillance study. J Med Internet Res. 22(4):e19016. PMID: 32287039. https://doi.org/10.2196/19016

Abd-alrazaq AA, Rababeh A, Alajlani M, Bewick BM, Househ M (2020c) The effectiveness and safety of using chatbots to improve mental health: a systematic review and meta-analysis. J Med Internet Res

Abdul A, Vermeulen J, Wang C, Lim BY, Kankanhalli MT (2018) Trajectories for explainable, accountable and intelligible systems: an HCI research Agenda. In: Proceedings of the 2018 CHI conference on human factors in computing systems; montreal QC, Canada: Association for computing machinery. p. Paper 582

Ai T, Yang Z, Hou H, Zhan C, Chen C, Lv W et al. (2019) Correlation of chest CT and RT-PCR testing in coronavirus disease 2019 (COVID-19) in China: a report of 1014 cases. Radiology. 0(0):200642. PMID: 32101510. https://doi.org/10.1148/radiol.2020200642

Alimadadi A, Aryal S, Manandhar I, Munroe PB, Joe B, Cheng X (2020) Artificial intelligence and machine learning to fight COVID-19. Physiol Genomics 52(4):200–2002. PMID: 32216577. https://doi.org/10.1152/physiolgenomics.00029.2020

Bogoch II, Watts A, Thomas-Bachli A, Huber C, Kraemer MUG, Khan K (2020) Pneumonia of unknown aetiology in Wuhan, China: potential for international spread via commercial air travel. J Travel Med 27(2). https://doi.org/10.1093/jtm/taaa008

Bryson L (2020) Cracking COVID-19: how BlueDot spots warning signs of pandemics | MaRS discovery district. In: MaRS discovery district, editor. MaRS 2020

Bullock J, Pham KH, Lam CSN, Luengo-Oroz M (2020) Mapping the landscape of artificial intelligence applications against COVID-19. arXiv preprint arXiv:200311336

Center of Diagnostics and Telemedicine (2020) Artificial intelligence in radiology [8 June 2020]. Available from: https://mosmed.ai/en/

Chen Y, Li L (2020) SARS-CoV-2: virus dynamics and host response. Lancet Infect Dis 20(5):515–516. https://doi.org/10.1016/S1473-3099(20)30235-8

Contreras I, Vehi J (2018) Artificial intelligence for diabetes management and decision support: literature review. J Med Internet Res 20(5):e10775. https://doi.org/10.2196/10775

del Rio C, Malani PN (2020) COVID-19—new insights on a rapidly changing epidemic. JAMA 323(14):1339–1340. https://doi.org/10.1001/jama.2020.3072

Deo RC (2015) Machine learning in medicine. Circulation 132(20):1920–30. PMID: 26572668. https://doi.org/10.1161/CIRCULATIONAHA.115.001593

Esteva A, Robicquet A, Ramsundar B, Kuleshov V, DePristo M, Chou K et al (2019) A guide to deep learning in healthcare. Nat Med 25(1):24–29. https://doi.org/10.1038/s41591-018-0316-z

European Commission (2020a) Liability for artificial intelligence and other emerging digital technologies

European Commission (2020b) White paper on artificial intelligence-A european approach to excellence and trust

Fan C, Zhang C, Yahja A, Mostafavi A (2019) Disaster city digital twin: a vision for integrating artificial and human intelligence for disaster management. Int J Inf Manage 102049. 27 Dec 2019. https://doi.org/10.1016/j.ijinfomgt.2019.102049

Feng C, Huang Z, Wang L, Chen X, Zhai Y, Zhu F et al (2020) A novel triage tool of artificial intelligence assisted diagnosis aid system for suspected COVID-19 pneumonia. In: Fever clinics. medRxiv. 2020:2020.03.19.20039099. https://doi.org/10.1101/2020.03.19.20039099

Fontanarosa PB, Bauchner H (2020) COVID-19—looking beyond tomorrow for health care and society. JAMA 323(19):1907–1908. https://doi.org/10.1001/jama.2020.6582

Goodman B, Flaxman S (2017) European Union regulations on algorithmic decision-making and a "right to explanation." AI Mag 38(3):50–57. https://doi.org/10.1609/aimag.v38i3.2741

Guo Q, Li M, Wang C, Wang P, Fang Z, Tan J et al (2019) Host and infectivity prediction of Wuhan 2019 novel coronavirus using deep learning algorithm. bioRxiv. 2020:2020.01.21.914044. https://doi.org/10.1101/2020.01.21.914044

HealthMap. About HealthMap (2020) [June 1, 2020]; Available from: https://www.healthmap.org/about/

Hosny A, Parmar C, Quackenbush J, Schwartz LH (2018) Aerts HJWL. Artificial intelligence in radiology. Nat Rev Cancer. 18(8):500–510. PMID: 29777175. https://doi.org/10.1038/s41568-018-0016-5

Imaging COVID-19 AI (2020) An european initiative for automated diagnosis and quantitative analysis of COVID-19 on imaging 2020 [08 June 2020]. Available from: https://imagingcovid19ai.eu/

International Telecommunication Union (2018) Focus group on "Artificial Intelligence for HEALTh" [08 June 2020]. Available from: https://www.itu.int/en/ITU-T/focusgroups/ai4h/Pages/default.aspx

Keeling MJ, Rohani P (2008) Modeling infectious diseases in humans and animals. Princeton University Press. ISBN: 9780691116174

Kong WH, Li Y, Peng MW, Kong DG, Yang XB, Wang L et al (2020) SARS-CoV-2 detection in patients with influenza-like illness. Nat Microbiol 5(5):675–678. PMID: 32265517. https://doi.org/10.1038/s41564-020-0713-1

Liao QV, Singh M, Zhang Y (2020) Bellamy RKE. Introduction to explainable ai. In: Extended abstracts of the 2020 CHI conference on human factors in computing systems. Association for Computing Machinery, Honolulu, HI, USA, pp 1–4

Long C, Xu H, Shen Q, Zhang X, Fan B, Wang C et al (2020) Diagnosis of the coronavirus disease (COVID-19): rRT-PCR or CT? Eur J Radiol. 126:108961, 01 May 2020. https://doi.org/10.1016/j.ejrad.2020.108961

Lopez-Rincon A, Tonda A, Mendoza-Maldonado L, Claassen E, Garssen J, Kraneveld AD (2020) Accurate identification of SARS-CoV-2 from viral genome sequences using deep learning. bioRxiv. 2020:2020.03.13.990242. https://doi.org/10.1101/2020.03.13.990242

Meng Z, Wang M, Song H, Guo S, Zhou Y, Li W et al (2020) Development and utilization of an intelligent application for aiding COVID-19 diagnosis. medRxiv. 2020:2020.03.18.20035816. https://doi.org/10.1101/2020.03.18.20035816

Morozov S (2020) How to visualAIze 5000 COVID CT scans daily with 15 minutes SLA? 2020 [cited 8 June 2020]. Available from: https://mosmed.ai/media/documents/How_to_visualAIze_5000_COVID_CT__en4.pdf

Naudé W (2020a) Artificial intelligence against COVID-19: an early review 1 June 2020. Available from: https://towardsdatascience.com/artificial-intelligence-against-covid-19-an-early-review-92a8360edaba

Naudé W (2020b) Artificial intelligence vs COVID-19: limitations, constraints and pitfalls. AI Soc 2020 Apr 28:1–5. PMID: 32346223. https://doi.org/10.1007/s00146-020-00978-0. Under the Creative Commons Attribution 4.0 International License (https://creativecommons.org/licenses/by/4.0/)

Niiler E (2020) An AI epidemiologist sent the first warnings of the Wuhan Virus 01 June 2020. Available from: https://www.wired.com/story/ai-epidemiologist-wuhan-public-health-warnings/

OECD (2020) Using artificial intelligence to help combat COVID-19 [03 June 2020]. Available from: https://read.oecd-ilibrary.org/view/?ref=130_130771-3jtyra9uoh&title=Using-artificial-intelligence-to-help-combat-COVID-19

Pandey R, Gautam V, Bhagat K, Sethi T (2020) A machine learning application for raising WASH awareness in the times of Covid-19 pandemic. arXiv preprint arXiv:200307074

Patel NV (2020) The best, and the worst, of the coronavirus dashboards [01 June 2020]. Available from: https://www.technologyreview.com/2020/03/06/905436/best-worst-coronavirus-dashboards/

Qatar Biomedical Research Institute (2020) QBRI insights: COVID-19: serological tests and neurological complications [08 June 2020]. Available from: https://www.hbku.edu.qa/en/news/serological-test-neurological

Randhawa GS, Soltysiak MPM, El Roz H, de Souza CPE, Hill KA, Kari L (2020) Machine learning using intrinsic genomic signatures for rapid classification of novel pathogens: COVID-19 case study. PLoS ONE 15(4):e0232391. https://doi.org/10.1371/journal.pone.0232391

Ribeiro MT, Singh M, Guestrin C (2016) "Why Should I Trust You?": Explaining the predictions of any classifier. In: Proceedings of the 22nd ACM SIGKDD international conference on knowledge discovery and data mining. Association for Computing Machinery, San Francisco, California, USA, pp 1135–1144

Russell S, Norvig P (2010) Artificial intelligence: a modern approach, 3rd edn. Prentice Hall, Upper Saddle River, New Jersey

Selbst AD, Powles J (2017) Meaningful information and the right to explanation. Int Data Priv Law 7(4):233–242. https://doi.org/10.1093/idpl/ipx022

Shi F, Wang J, Shi J, Wu Z, Wang Q, Tang Z et al (2020) Review of artificial intelligence techniques in imaging data acquisition, segmentation and diagnosis for COVID-19. IEEE Rev Biomed Eng 2020 Apr 16. PMID: 32305937. https://doi.org/10.1109/rbme.2020.2987975

Tahamtan A, Ardebili A (2020) Real-time RT-PCR in COVID-19 detection: issues affecting the results. Expert Rev Mol Diagn 20(5):453–454. PMID: 32297805. https://doi.org/10.1080/14737159.2020.1757437

van Hartskamp M, Consoli S, Verhaegh W, Petkovic M, van de Stolpe A (2019) Artificial intelligence in clinical health care applications: viewpoint. Interact J Med Res 8(2):e12100. PMID: 30950806. https://doi.org/10.2196/12100

VanBerlo B, Ross M (2020) Investigation of explainable predictions of COVID-19 infection from chest X-rays with machine learning. Artif Intell Lab [08 June 2020]. Available from: https://towardsdatascience.com/investigation-of-explainable-predictions-of-covid-19-infection-from-chest-x-rays-with-machine-cb370f46af1d

Varshney KR (2019) Trustworthy machine learning and artificial intelligence. XRDS: Crossroads. ACM Mag Students 25(3):26–29

Wachter S, Mittelstadt B, Floridi L (2017) Why a right to explanation of automated decision-making does not exist in the general data protection regulation. Inter Data Privac Law 7(2):76–99. https://doi.org/10.1093/idpl/ipx005

Wang Y, Hu M, Li Q, Zhang X-P, Zhai G, Yao N (2020a) Abnormal respiratory patterns classifier may contribute to large-scale screening of people infected with COVID-19 in an accurate and unobtrusive manner. arXiv preprint arXiv:200205534

Wang Z, Li L, Yan J, Yao Y (2020b) Evaluating the traditional Chinese medicine (TCM) officially recommended in China for COVID-19 using ontology-based side-effect prediction framework (OSPF) and deep learning. Preprints.org; 2020

World Health Organization (2020) Coronavirus disease 2019 (COVID-19): situation report-136

Wynants L, Van Calster B, Collins GS, Riley RD, Heinze G, Schuit E et al. (2020) Prediction models for diagnosis and prognosis of covid-19: systematic review and critical appraisal. BMJ 369:m1328. https://doi.org/10.1136/bmj.m1328

Yang P, Wang X (2020) COVID-19: a new challenge for human beings. Cell Mol Immunol 17(5):555–557, 01 May 2020. https://doi.org/10.1038/s41423-020-0407-x.

Printed in the United States
by Baker & Taylor Publisher Services